## POCKET GUIDE TO

# Fluid, Electrolyte, and Acid-Base Balance

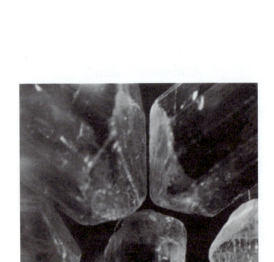

Calcium phosphate crystals.

POCKET GUIDE TO

# Fluid, Electrolyte, and Acid-Base Balance

## Mima M. Horne, R.N., M.S., C.D.E.

Diabetes Clinical Nurse Specialist
New Hanover Regional Medical Center
Adjunct Faculty
University of North Carolina at Wilmington
Wilmington, North Carolina

## Ursula Easterday Heitz, R.N., M.S.N.

Nursing Consultant
Nashville, Tennessee

## Pamela L. Swearingen, R.N.

Special Project Editor
Denver, Colorado

With contributions by
**Karen S. Webber, R.N., M.N.**
Assistant Professor, School of Nursing
Memorial University of Newfoundland
St. John's, Newfoundland

**Third Edition**

17 illustrations

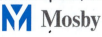 Mosby

St. Louis  Baltimore  Boston
Carlsbad  Chicago  Naples  New York  Philadelphia  Portland
London  Madrid  Mexico City  Singapore  Sydney  Tokyo  Toronto  Wiesbaden

Vice President and Publisher: Nancy L. Coon
Editor: Loren Wilson
Developmental Editor: Brian Dennison
Project Manager: Patricia Tannian
Senior Production Editor: Suzanne C. Fannin
Book Design Manager: Gail Morey Hudson
Cover Designer: Teresa Breckwoldt
Manufacturing Supervisor: Karen Lewis
Cover Photograph: © Goivaux Communication/Phototake NYC

A NOTE TO THE READER:
The author and publisher have made every attempt to check dosages and
nursing content for accuracy. Because the science of pharmacology is
continually advancing, our knowledge base continues to expand. Therefore we
recommend that the reader always check product information for changes in
dosage or administration before administering any medication. This is
particularly important with new or rarely used drugs.

Printed in the United States of America

Composition by Graphic World, Inc.
Printing/binding by R.R. Donnelley & Sons Company

Mosby–Year Book, Inc.
11830 Westline Industrial Drive
St. Louis, Missouri 63146

**Library of Congress Cataloging in Publication Data**

Horne, Mima M.
    Pocket guide to fluid, electrolyte, and acid-base balance / Mima
M. Horne, Ursula Easterday Heitz, Pamela L. Swearingen ; with
contributions by Karen S. Webber.—3rd ed.
        p.      cm.
    Includes bibliographical references and index.
    ISBN 0-8151-4663-9
    1. Body fluid disorders—Nursing—Handbooks, manuals, etc.
2. Water-electrolyte imbalances—Nursing—Handbooks, manuals, etc.
3. Acid-base imbalances—Nursing—Handbooks, manuals, etc.
I. Heitz, Ursula Easterday. II. Swearingen, Pamela L. III. Title.
    [DNLM: 1. Body Fluids—handbooks. 2. Body Fluids—nurses'
instruction. 3. Water-Electrolyte Imbalance—handbooks. 4. Water
-Electrolyte Imbalance—nurses' instruction. 5. Acid-Base
Imbalance—handbooks. 6. Acid-Base Imbalance—nurses' instruction.
QU 39 H815p 1997]
RC630.P63 1997
616.3′9—dc20
DNLM/DLC
for Library of Congress                                96-10272
                                                            CIP

98   99   00   /   9   8   7   6   5   4   3   2

# Preface

*Pocket Guide to Fluid, Electrolyte, and Acid-Base Balance,*
3rd edition, was developed to provide nursing students and
practicing nurses with quick, practical information on pathophysiology, assessment, diagnostic tests, collaborative management,
nursing diagnoses, and nursing interventions for patients with fluid,
electrolyte, and acid-base imbalances. Given its portable size, the
book is unique in that its coverage of content is both extensive and
concise. The organization of the second edition has been retained,
including the use of unit subdivisions to facilitate retrieval of
content. Each disorder is presented in a consistent format to
enhance utility in the clinical environment. The outline format,
boldface headings, use of color, and illustrations reinforce the
book's clarity and further enhance its usability. In addition, all
efforts have been made to ensure the level of presentation is as easy
to understand as possible. This is especially important in content
related to fluid, electrolyte, and acid-base balance because the
material often is presented in a way that makes comprehension
difficult.

Nurses can use this reference for either of two purposes:
1. To identify a patient's specific fluid, electrolyte, or acid-base
   disturbance in Unit II and review the nursing diagnoses and
   care for that specific disturbance.
2. To identify the medical diagnosis (e.g., diabetic ketoacidosis)
   in Unit III and review the list of fluid, electrolyte, and
   acid-base disturbances associated with that particular disorder (i.e., hypokalemia, hypovolemia, hypophosphatemia)
   and then refer back to the chapters in Unit II that cover these
   disturbances in detail.

This edition has been thoroughly revised and updated with the
addition of content relevant to both the critical care patient and the
patient in the subacute setting (i.e., homecare). Wherever possible,
we have expanded content related to the pediatric and geriatric
patients. Although this third edition includes more detailed
information about infants and children, the reader is advised that all
numbers refer to the adult unless otherwise specified. As before, the
appendices are unusually detailed. They include common abbre-

viations, a glossary of terms, and normal values for laboratory tests discussed in the text, as well as tables describing the effects of age on fluid, electrolyte, and acid-base balance.

We wish to thank our contributor, Karen S. Weber, for a job well done. We also thank Roberta J. Secrest, Ph.D., Pharm.D., R.Ph; Senior Associate Scientist, Marion Merrell Dow Research Institute, Cincinnati, Ohio; and Marianne Saunorus Baird, R.N., M.N., CCRN, Clinical Nurse Specialist, St. Joseph's Hospital of Atlanta, Atlanta, Georgia, for their many helpful suggestions on the third edition.

*Pocket Guide to Fluid, Electrolyte, and Acid-Base Balance* was written to supplement medical-surgical textbooks and assumes the reader has a basic understanding of pathophysiology and assessment. The book also serves as a resource for practicing nurses and academicians. Our primary goals are to make information about fluids, electrolytes, acids, bases, and related topics understandable and to facilitate application of that information to patient care. Reviewers indicate that we have achieved these objectives, and we welcome comments and suggestions from our readers so that we may enhance the book's usefulness in future editions.

*Mima M. Horne*

*Ursula Easterday Heitz*

*Pamela L. Swearingen*

# Brief Contents

Unit I    Basic Principles, 1

1    Overview of Fluid and Electrolyte Balance, 3
2    Regulation of Vascular Volume and Extracellular Fluid Osmolality, 14
3    Fluid Gains and Losses, 23
4    Nursing Assessment of the Patient at Risk, 27
5    Laboratory Assessment of Fluid, Electrolyte, and Acid-Base Balance, 35

Unit II    Disorders of Fluid, Electrolyte, and Acid-Base Balance, 47

6    Disorders of Fluid Balance, 49
7    Disorders of Sodium Balance, 87
8    Disorders of Potassium Balance, 95
9    Disorders of Calcium Balance, 107
10    Disorders of Phosphorus Balance, 118
11    Disorders of Magnesium Balance, 130
12    Overview of Acid-Base Balance, 140
13    Respiratory Acidosis, 153
14    Respiratory Alkalosis, 165
15    Metabolic Acidosis, 170
16    Metabolic Alkalosis, 179
17    Mixed Acid-Base Disorders, 186

Unit III    Clinical Conditions Associated with Fluid, Electrolyte, and Acid-Base Imbalance, 191

18    Gastrointestinal Disorders, 193
19    Surgical Disturbances, 201
20    Endocrinologic Disorders, 204

21  Cardiac Disorders, 218

22  Renal Failure, 221

23  Acute Pancreatitis, 230

24  Hepatic Failure, 233

25  Burns, 237

26  Providing Nutritional Support, 245

Selected References, 265

Appendices

A  Abbreviations Used in This Manual, 270

B  Glossary, 274

C  Effects of Age on Fluid, Electrolyte, and Acid-Base Balance, 281

D  Laboratory Tests Discussed in This Manual (Normal Values), 284

# Contents

Unit I    Basic Principles, 1

1    Overview of Fluid and Electrolyte Balance, 3

Composition of body fluids, 3
  Water, 3
  Solutes, 4
Fluid compartments, 6
  Intracellular fluid, 6
  Extracellular fluid, 6
Factors that affect movement of water and solutes, 8
  Membranes, 8
  Transport processes, 8
  Concentration of body fluids, 11

2    Regulation of Vascular Volume and Extracellular Fluid
     Osmolality, 14

Regulation of vascular volume, 14
  Sympathetic nervous system, 18
  Renin-angiotensin, 19
  Aldosterone, 19
  Atrial natriuretic factor, 19
  Antidiuretic hormone and thirst, 20
Regulation of extracellular fluid osmolality, 20
  Defense of brain cell volume, 22

3    Fluid Gains and Losses, 23

Fluid gains, 23
  Oxidative metabolism, 23
  Oral fluids, 24
  Solid food, 24
  Fluid therapy, 24
Fluid losses, 24
  Kidneys, 24
  Skin, 25
  Lungs, 26
  Gastrointestinal tract, 26
  Additional losses, 26
  Third-space losses, 26

4   Nursing Assessment of the Patient at Risk, 27
    Nursing history, 27
        Physiologic, 27
        Developmental, 27
        Psychologic, 28
        Spiritual, 28
        Sociocultural, 28
    Clinical assessment, 28
        Daily weights, 28
        Intake and output, 29
    Hemodynamic monitoring, 29
    Vital signs, 30
        Body temperature, 30
        Respiratory rate and depth, 31
        Heart rate/pulses, 31
        Blood pressure, 31
    Physical assessment, 32
        Integument, 32
        Cardiovascular system, 32
        Neurologic system, 33
        Gastrointestinal system, 34

5   Laboratory Assessment of Fluid, Electrolyte, and
    Acid-Base Balance, 35
    Tests to evaluate fluid status, 35
        Serum osmolality, 35
        Hematocrit, 36
        Urea nitrogen, 36
        Urine osmolality, 37
        Urine specific gravity, 38
        Urine sodium, 39
    Tests to evaluate electrolyte balance, 39
    Tests to evaluate acid-base balance, 40
        Arterial blood gases, 40
        Carbon dioxide content or total carbon dioxide, 40
        Anion gap, 41
        Urine pH, 42
        Lactic acid, 44
    Related tests, 44
        Creatinine, 44
        Serum albumin, 44

Unit II    Disorders of Fluid, Electrolyte,
          and Acid-Base Balance, 47

6    Disorders of Fluid Balance, 49
     Hypovolemia, 49
          Assessment, 49
          Diagnostic tests, 52
          Collaborative management, 53
          Nursing diagnoses and interventions, 65
          Patient-family teaching guidelines, 67
     Hypervolemia, 68
          Assessment, 68
          Diagnostic tests, 68
          Collaborative management, 69
          Nursing diagnoses and interventions, 70
          Patient-family teaching guidelines, 72
     Edema formation, 73
          Assessment, 74
          Collaborative management, 75
          Diuretic therapy, 75
          Complications of diuretic therapy, 75
     Intravenous fluid therapy, 80
          Commonly prescribed intravenous fluids, 81

7    Disorders of Sodium Balance, 87
     Sodium changes, 87
     Hyponatremia, 88
          Assessment, 88
          Diagnostic tests, 89
          Collaborative management, 89
          Nursing diagnoses and interventions, 90
          Patient-family teaching guidelines, 91
     Hypernatremia, 91
          Assessment, 91
          Diagnostic tests, 92
          Collaborative management, 93
          Nursing diagnoses and interventions, 93
          Patient-family teaching guidelines, 94

8    Disorders of Potassium Balance, 95
     Hypokalemia, 96
          Assessment, 96

Diagnostic tests, 97
Collaborative management, 97
Nursing diagnoses and interventions, 99
Patient-family teaching guidelines, 101
Hyperkalemia, 102
Assessment, 102
Diagnostic tests, 103
Collaborative management, 103
Nursing diagnoses and interventions, 104
Patient-family teaching guidelines, 106

**9  Disorders of Calcium Balance, 107**

Hypocalcemia, 108
Assessment, 108
Diagnostic tests, 109
Collaborative management, 109
Nursing diagnoses and interventions, 110
Patient-family teaching guidelines, 112
Hypercalcemia, 113
Assessment, 113
Diagnostic tests, 114
Collaborative management, 114
Nursing diagnoses and interventions, 115
Patient-family teaching guidelines, 116

**10  Disorders of Phosphorus Balance, 118**

Hypophosphatemia, 119
Assessment, 119
Diagnostic tests, 121
Collaborative management, 121
Nursing diagnoses and interventions, 122
Patient-family teaching guidelines, 124
Hyperphosphatemia, 125
Assessment, 125
Diagnostic tests, 126
Collaborative management, 126
Nursing diagnoses and interventions, 127
Patient-family teaching guidelines, 129

**11  Disorders of Magnesium Balance, 130**

Hypomagnesemia, 131
Assessment, 131

Diagnostic tests, 132
Collaborative management, 133
Nursing diagnoses and interventions, 133
Patient-family teaching guidelines, 136
Hypermagnesemia, 136
Assessment, 136
Diagnostic tests, 137
Collaborative management, 137
Nursing diagnoses and interventions, 138
Patient-family teaching guidelines, 139

**12    Overview of Acid-Base Balance, 140**

Buffer system responses, 140
Buffers, 140
Respiratory system, 141
Renal system, 141
Blood gas values, 142
Arterial blood gas analysis, 142
Step-by-step guide to arterial blood gas analysis, 144
Arterial-venous difference, 149

**13    Respiratory Acidosis, 153**

Acute respiratory acidosis, 153
Assessment, 153
Diagnostic tests, 155
Collaborative management, 155
Nursing diagnoses and interventions, 156
Chronic respiratory acidosis (compensated), 160
Assessment, 160
Diagnostic tests, 161
Collaborative management, 162
Nursing diagnoses and interventions, 162

**14    Respiratory Alkalosis, 165**

Acute respiratory alkalosis, 165
Assessment, 165
Diagnostic tests, 166
Collaborative management, 167
Nursing diagnoses and interventions, 167
Chronic respiratory alkalosis, 168
Assessment, 168
Diagnostic tests, 168

Collaborative management, 169
Nursing diagnoses and interventions, 169

15   Metabolic Acidosis, 170
Acute metabolic acidosis, 170
   Assessment, 170
   Diagnostic tests, 172
   Collaborative management, 173
   Nursing diagnoses and interventions, 175
Chronic metabolic acidosis, 175
   Assessment, 175
   Diagnostic tests, 175
   Collaborative management, 177
   Nursing diagnoses and interventions, 177

16   Metabolic Alkalosis, 179
Acute metabolic alkalosis, 179
   Assessment, 179
   Diagnostic tests, 181
   Collaborative management, 181
   Nursing diagnoses and interventions, 182
Chronic metabolic alkalosis, 183
   Assessment, 183
   Diagnostic tests, 184
   Collaborative management, 184
   Nursing diagnoses and interventions, 185

17   Mixed Acid-Base Disorders, 186
Mixed acid-base disorders, 186
   Case study one, 186
   Case study two, 187
   Case study three, 188
   Case study four, 188

Unit III   Clinical Conditions Associated with Fluid,
           Electrolyte, and Acid-Base Imbalance, 191
18   Gastrointestinal Disorders, 193
Loss of upper gastrointestinal contents, 193
   Saliva, 193
   Gastric juices, 195
   Gastric suction, 195

Potential fluid, electrolyte, and acid-base disturbances
with loss of upper gastrointestinal contents, 196
Loss of lower gastrointestinal contents, 197
Pancreatic juice, 198
Bile, 198
Intestinal secretions, 198
Diarrhea, 198
Bowel obstruction, 199
Potential fluid, electrolyte, and acid-base disturbances
with loss of lower gastrointestinal contents, 200

**19   Surgical Disturbances, 201**
Preoperative factors, 201
Intraoperative factors, 202
Postoperative factors, 202

**20   Endocrinologic Disorders, 204**
Diabetic ketoacidosis, 204
Potential fluid, electrolyte, and acid-base disturbances, 205
Hyperosmolar hyperglycemic nonketotic syndrome, 206
Potential fluid, electrolyte, and acid-base
disturbances, 207
Diabetes insipidus, 211
Potential fluid, electrolyte, and acid-base
disturbances, 211
Syndrome of inappropriate antidiuretic hormone, 215
Potential fluid, electrolyte, and acid-base
disturbances, 215
Acute adrenal insufficiency, 216
Potential fluid, electrolyte, and acid-base
disturbances, 216

**21   Cardiac Disorders, 218**
Congestive heart failure and pulmonary edema, 218
Potential fluid, electrolyte, and acid-base
disturbances, 219
Cardiogenic shock, 219
Potential fluid, electrolyte, and acid-base
disturbances, 220

**22   Renal Failure, 221**
Potential fluid, electrolyte, and acid-base disturbances, 226

23   Acute Pancreatitis, 230
         Potential fluid, electrolyte, and acid-base
            disturbances, 230

24   Hepatic Failure, 233
         Potential fluid, electrolyte, and acid-base
            disturbances, 234

25   Burns, 237
         Potential fluid, electrolyte, and acid-base
            disturbances, 242

26   Providing Nutritional Support, 245
     Nutritional assessment, 245
         Nutritional history, 245
         Physical assessment, 246
         Anthropometric data, 246
         Height, 246
         Weight, 246
         Body mass index, 247
         Triceps skin fold thickness, 247
         Biochemical data, 247
         Estimating nutritional requirements, 248
     Nutritional support modalities, 250
         Enteral nutrition, 250
         Parenteral nutrition, 256
     Transitional feeding, 261
         Potential fluid, electrolyte, and acid-base
            disturbances, 261
         Fluid imbalances, 261
         Electrolyte imbalances, 263
         Acid-base imbalance, 264

Selected References, 265

Appendices
A    Abbreviations Used in This Manual, 270
B    Glossary, 274
C    Effects of Age on Fluid, Electrolyte, and Acid-Base
     Balance, 281
D    Laboratory Tests Discussed in This Manual (Normal
     Values), 284

# BASIC
# PRINCIPLES

I

# Overview of Fluid and Electrolyte Balance

1

The cell is the fundamental functioning unit of the human body. For body cells to perform their individual physiologic tasks, a stable environment is necessary, including maintenance of a steady supply of nutrients and the continuous removal of metabolic wastes. Careful regulation of body fluids helps ensure a stable internal environment.

## Composition of Body Fluids

All body fluids are dilute solutions of water and dissolved substances (solutes).

### Water

Water is the major constituent of the human body. The average adult male is approximately 60% water by weight, and the average female is approximately 55% water by weight. Factors that affect body water include:

1. **Fat cells:** They contain little water, thus body water decreases with increasing body fat.
2. **Age:** As a rule, body water decreases with increasing age. Premature infants may be as much as 80% water by weight, whereas the full-term infant is approximately 70% water by weight. By the age of 6 months to 1 year, body water decreases to approximately 60%, with little further reduction throughout childhood. The older adult may be 45% to 55% water by weight. The percentage of water decreases as muscle mass declines in the elderly. See Table 1-1.
3. **Female gender:** Women have proportionately less body water because they have proportionately greater body fat.

**Table 1-1**   Changes in total body water with age

| Age | Kilogram Weight (%) |
|---|---|
| Premature infant | 80 |
| 3 mo | 70 |
| 6 mo | 60 |
| 1-2 yr | 59 |
| 11-16 yr | 58 |
| Adult | 58-60 |
| Obese adult | 40-50 |
| Emaciated adult | 70-75 |

From Gröer MW: *Physiology and pathophysiology of the body fluids,* ed 1, St Louis, 1981, Mosby.

## Solutes

In addition to water, body fluids contain two types of dissolved substances (solutes): electrolytes and nonelectrolytes.

1. **Electrolytes:** Substances that dissociate (separate) in solution and will conduct an electric current. Electrolytes dissociate into positive and negative ions and are measured by their capacity to combine with each other (milliequivalents/liter [mEq/L]) or by their molecular weight in grams (millimoles/liter [mmol/L]). The number of cations and anions, as measured in milliequivalents, in solution is always equal.
   - *Cations:* Ions that develop a positive charge in solution. The primary extracellular cation is sodium ($Na^+$), whereas the primary intracellular cation is potassium ($K^+$). A pump system exists in the wall of body cells that pumps sodium out and potassium in.
   - *Anions:* Ions that develop a negative charge in solution. The primary extracellular anion is chloride ($Cl^-$), whereas the primary intracellular anion is phosphate ion ($PO_4^{3-}$). Because the electrolyte content of the plasma and interstitial fluids is essentially the same (Table 1-2), plasma electrolyte values reflect the composition of the extracellular fluid, which is composed of intravascular and interstitial fluids (see "Fluid Compartments," p. 6). However, plasma electrolyte values do not necessarily reflect the electrolyte composition of the intracellular fluid. Understanding the difference

**Table 1-2** Primary constituents of body fluid compartments

| Compartment | $Na^+$ (mEq/L) | $K^+$ (mEq/L) | $Cl^-$ (mEq/L) | $HCO_3^-$ (mEq/L) | $PO_4^{3-}$ (mEq/L) |
|---|---|---|---|---|---|
| Intravascular (plasma) | 142 | 4.5 | 104 | 24 | 2 |
| Interstitial | 145 | 4.4 | 117 | 27 | 2.3 |
| Intracellular (skeletal muscle cell) | 12 | 150 | 4 | 12 | 40 |
| Transcellular | | | | | |
| Gastric juice | 60 | 7 | 100 | 0 | — |
| Pancreatic juice | 130 | 7 | 60 | 100 | — |
| Sweat | 45 | 5 | 58 | 0 | — |

This is a partial list. Other constituents include calcium ion $Ca^{2+}$, magnesium ion $Mg^{2+}$, sulfates, proteinates, and organic acids.
NOTE: Values given are average ones. (Modified from Rose BD: *Clinical physiology of acid-base and electrolyte disorders,* ed 3, New York, 1989, McGraw-Hill Book.)

between these two compartments is important in anticipating the types of imbalances that can occur with certain disorders such as tissue trauma or acid-base imbalances. In these situations, electrolytes may be released from or move into or out of the cells, significantly altering plasma electrolyte values. See discussions of potassium balance, Chapter 8, and phosphorus balance, Chapter 10.

2. **Nonelectrolytes:** Substances such as glucose and urea that do not dissociate in solution and are measured by weight (milligrams per 100 ml [mg/dl]). Other clinically important nonelectrolytes include *creatinine* and *bilirubin.*

# Fluid Compartments

Body fluids are distributed between two major fluid compartments: the intracellular compartment and the extracellular compartment (Figure 1-1).

## Intracellular Fluid

Intracellular fluid (ICF) is the fluid contained within the cells. In the adult, approximately two thirds of the body's fluid is intracellular, equalling approximately 27 L in the average (70 kg) adult male. In contrast, only half of an infant's body fluid is intracellular.

## Extracellular Fluid

Extracellular fluid (ECF) is the fluid outside the cells. The *relative* size of ECF decreases with advancing age. In the newborn, approximately half the body fluid is contained within ECF. After 1 year of age, the *relative* volume of ECF decreases to approximately one third of the total volume. This equals approximately 15 L in the average (70 kg) adult male. ECF is further divided into the following:

1. **Interstitial fluid (ISF):** The fluid surrounding the cells, equal to approximately 11 to 12 L in the adult. Lymph fluid is included in the interstitial volume. Relative to body size, the volume of ISF is approximately twice as great in the newborn as in the adult.

2. **Intravascular fluid (IVF):** The fluid contained within the blood vessels. The *relative* volume of IVF is similar in adults and children. Average adult blood volume is approximately 5 to 6 L, of which about 3 L is plasma. The remaining 2 to

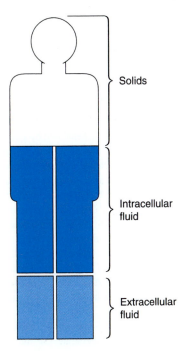

**Figure 1-1**
Comparison of intracellular fluid to extracellular fluid.

3 L consist of red blood cells (RBCs, or erythrocytes), which transport oxygen and act as important body buffers; white blood cells (WBCs, or leukocytes); and platelets. Functions of the blood include:

- Delivery of nutrients (e.g., glucose and oxygen) to the tissues
- Transport of waste products to the kidneys and lungs
- Delivery of antibodies and WBCs to sites of infection
- Transport of hormones to their sites of action
- Circulation of body heat

3. **Transcellular fluid (TCF):** The fluid contained within specialized cavities of the body. Examples of TCF include cerebrospinal, pericardial, pleural, synovial, and intraocular fluids, and digestive secretions. At any given time, TCF is

approximately 1 L. However, large amounts of fluid may move into and out of the transcellular space each day. For example, the gastrointestinal tract normally secretes and reabsorbs up to 6 to 8 L per day.

# Factors that Affect Movement of Water and Solutes
## Membranes

Each of the fluid compartments is separated by a selectively permeable membrane that permits the movement of water and some solutes. Although small molecules such as urea and water move freely among all compartments, certain substances move less readily. Plasma proteins, for example, are restricted to the IVF, owing to the low permeability of the capillary membrane to large molecules. Selective permeability of membranes helps maintain the unique composition of each compartment while allowing for the movement of nutrients from the plasma to the cells and the movement of waste products out of the cells and eventually into the plasma. The body's semipermeable membranes include:

1. **Cell membranes:** Separate ICF from ISF and are composed of lipids and protein.
2. **Capillary membranes:** Separate IVF from ISF.
3. **Epithelial membranes:** Separate ISF and IVF from TCF. Examples of epithelial membranes include the mucosal epithelium of the stomach and intestines, the synovial membrane, and the renal tubules.

## Transport Processes

In addition to membrane selectivity, the movement of water and solutes is determined by several transport processes.

1. **Diffusion:** The random movement of particles in all directions through a solution or gas. Particles move from an area of high concentration to an area of low concentration along a concentration gradient. The energy for diffusion is produced by thermal energy. An example of diffusion is the movement of oxygen from the alveoli of the lung to the blood of the pulmonary capillaries. Diffusion also may occur because of changes in electric potential across the membrane. Cations will follow anions and vice versa. See the box on p. 9 for a list of factors that increase diffusion (opposite factors will act to reduce diffusion).

## Factors that Increase Diffusion*

- Increased temperature
- Increased concentration of the particle
- Decreased size or molecular weight of the particle
- Increased surface area available for diffusion
- Decreased distance across which the particle mass must diffuse

*NOTE: Opposite factors will act to reduce diffusion.

Cell walls are composed of sheets of lipids with many minute protein pores. Substances may diffuse across the cell wall under the following conditions:

- If they are small enough to pass through the protein pores (e.g., water and urea): This is termed *simple diffusion.*
- If they are lipid soluble (e.g., oxygen and carbon dioxide): This is another example of simple diffusion.
- By means of a carrier substance: This is termed *facilitated diffusion.* Large lipid-insoluble substance such as glucose must diffuse into the cell via a carrier substance. Glucose, for example, combines with a carrier on the outside of the cell to become lipid soluble. Once inside the cell, glucose breaks away from the carrier and the carrier is then free to facilitate diffusion of additional glucose.

As with simple diffusion, facilitated diffusion requires the presence of a concentration gradient that favors diffusion. The rate of facilitated diffusion, however, depends on the availability of the carrier substance. If there is a large concentration gradient (i.e., the difference between the areas of high and low concentration is great), the carrier can become saturated (used up), and diffusion will decrease despite the presence of a favorable concentration gradient. Glucose will move into the cell, for example, only if there is a favorable concentration gradient and an available carrier substance.

2. **Active transport:** Simple diffusion will not occur in the absence of a favorable electric or concentration gradient. Energy is required for a substance to move from an area of lesser or equal concentration to an area of equal or higher

concentration. This is termed *active transport,* and like facilitated diffusion, it depends on the availability of carrier substances. Many important solutes are transported actively across cell membranes, including sodium, potassium, hydrogen, glucose, and amino acids. The renal tubules, for example, depend on active transport to reabsorb all the glucose filtered by the glomeruli to enable excretion of urine that is glucose-free. As with facilitated diffusion, the carriers can become overwhelmed or saturated. In the case of glucose within the renal tubule, saturation occurs when the blood sugar exceeds approximately 180 to 200 mg/dl. Active transport is vital for maintaining the unique composition of both the ECF and ICF.

3. **Filtration:** The movement of water and solutes from an area of high hydrostatic pressure to an area of low hydrostatic pressure. *Hydrostatic pressure* is the pressure created by the weight of fluid. Filtration is important in directing fluid out of the arterial end of the capillaries. It is also the force that enables the kidneys to filter 180 L of plasma a day.

4. **Osmosis:** The movement of water across a semipermeable membrane from an area of lower solute concentration to an area of higher solute concentration. Osmosis can occur across any membrane when solute concentrations on either side of the membrane change. The following are terms that are associated with osmosis:

   - *Osmotic pressure:* The amount of hydrostatic pressure required to stop the osmotic flow of water.
   - *Oncotic pressure:* The osmotic pressure exerted by colloids (proteins). Albumin, for example, exerts oncotic pressure within the blood vessels and helps hold the water content of the blood in the intravascular space.
   - *Osmotic diuresis:* Increased urine output caused by substances such as mannitol, glucose, or contrast media, which are excreted in the urine and reduce renal water reabsorption. For example, an osmotic diuresis occurs in uncontrolled diabetes mellitus because of the presence of excess glucose in the renal tubule. When the blood sugar is within normal range, all the glucose that is filtered by the kidney is reabsorbed (saved) via active transport. In hyperglycemia (blood sugar >180 to 200 mg/dl), the kidneys' ability to reabsorb glucose is overwhelmed (i.e.,

the carrier substance becomes saturated). The glucose that is not reabsorbed remains in the tubule and acts osmotically to hold water that otherwise would be reabsorbed. The net result is *glucosuria* and *polyuria.*

## Concentration of Body Fluids

1. **Osmolality:** As discussed previously, changes in the concentration of body fluids affect the movement of water among fluid compartments by osmosis. The measure of a solution's ability to create osmotic pressure and thus affect the movement of water is termed *osmolality.* Osmolality also may be described as a measure of the concentration of body fluids (the ratio of solutes to water) because it is reported in milliosmoles (1 one thousandth of an osmole) per kilogram of water (mOsm/kg). One osmole contains $6 \times 10^{23}$ particles. *Osmolarity,* another term used to describe the concentration of solutions, reflects the number of particles in a liter of solution and is measured in milliosmoles per liter (mOsm/L). Because body fluids are relatively dilute, the difference between their osmolality and osmolarity is small, and the terms often are used interchangeably. Osmolality is the measure used to evaluate serum and urine in clinical practice.

   Changes in extracellular osmolality may result in changes in both extracellular and intracellular fluid volume:

   *Decreased ECF osmolality → movement of water from the ECF to the ICF*

   *Increased ECF osmolality → movement of water from the ICF to the ECF*

   Water will continue to move until the osmolality of the two compartments reaches equilibrium. This is the rationale for using intravenous mannitol in the treatment of cerebral edema. Mannitol increases the osmolality of the ECF, promoting the movement of water out of the cerebral cells, thereby reducing cellular swelling.

   Osmolality of the ECF may be determined by measuring serum osmolality (see Chapter 5). Sodium is the primary determinant of ECF osmolality. Because it is limited primarily to the ECF, sodium acts to hold water in that compartment. Potassium helps maintain the volume of ICF, and the plasma proteins help maintain the volume of the intravascular space (IVS).

2. **Tonicity:** Small molecules, like urea, that readily cross all membranes quickly equilibrate among compartments and have little effect on the movement of water. These small molecules are termed *ineffective osmoles.* In contrast, sodium, glucose, and mannitol are examples of *effective osmoles;* they do not cross the cell membrane quickly and will, therefore, affect the movement of water. Thus *effective osmolality* (i.e., osmolality that will cause water to move from one compartment to another) is dependent not only on the number of solutes but also on the permeability of the membrane to these solutes. *Tonicity* is another term for effective osmolality.

   ■ *Isotonic solutions:* Those that have the same effective osmolality as body fluids (approximately 280 to 300 mOsm/kg). An example is normal saline—0.9% sodium chloride (NaCl) solution.

   ■ *Hypotonic solutions:* Those that have an effective osmolality less than body fluids. An example is 0.45% NaCl solution.

   ■ *Hypertonic solutions:* Those that have an effective osmolality greater than body fluids. An example is 3% NaCl solution.

   *Clinical hypotonicity* occurs when there is an abnormal gain in water or loss of sodium-rich fluids with replacement by

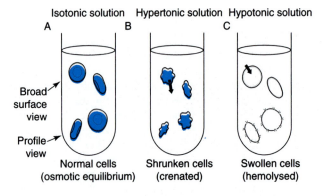

Isotonic solution   Hypertonic solution   Hypotonic solution

A   B   C

Broad surface view

Profile view

Normal cells (osmotic equilibrium)   Shrunken cells (crenated)   Swollen cells (hemolysed)

Figure 1-2
Effect of osmotic pressure on the cells.

water only. *Clinical hypertonicity* may develop because of loss of water (e.g., diabetes insipidus), loss of hypotonic body fluids (e.g., sweating, diarrhea), or gain of effective osmoles (e.g., hyperglycemia or administration of hypertonic NaCl, sodium bicarbonate, or mannitol). Hyperosmolality *without* hypertonicity (does not cause cellular dehydration) occurs with the ingestion of methyl alcohol or ethylene glycol or in renal failure secondary to retention of urea. See Figure 1-2 for a depiction of osmotic pressure on the cells.

# Regulation of Vascular Volume and Extracellular Fluid Osmolality

2

To provide an optimal environment for the body's cells, the composition, concentration, and volume of the extracellular fluid (ECF) are regulated by a combination of renal, metabolic, and neurologic functions. The ECF is continuously altered and then modified as the body reacts with its surrounding environment. In contrast, the intracellular fluid (ICF) is protected by the ECF and remains relatively stable, ensuring normal cellular function. Because the primary constituents of the ECF are water and sodium (and sodium's accompanying anions), their regulation is crucial for maintaining the volume and concentration of the ECF (Figures 2-1, 2-2, and 2-3). Regulation of the composition of the ECF depends on the regulation of the individual electrolytes (see Chapters 7 through 11).

## Regulation of Vascular Volume

Large fluctuations can occur in the volume of the interstitial portion of the ECF without markedly affecting body functions. This is especially true if the changes occur slowly. Individuals with cirrhosis, for example, often are able to tolerate significant amounts of ascitic fluid. The vascular portion of the ECF is less tolerant of change and must be maintained carefully to ensure that the tissues receive an adequate supply of nutrients and continuous removal of metabolic wastes without compromising the cardiovascular system. The portion of the intravascular fluid that effectively perfuses tissues is termed the *effective circulating volume (ECV)*.

Changes in the ECV are sensed by specialized receptors located in the carotid sinuses, aortic arch, cardiac artria, and renal vessels. These volume receptors do not measure total volume but rather respond to changes in pressure via changes in stretch in the arterial or atrial wall. Increases in ECV cause an increase in blood pressure and thus stretch at these receptors. In contrast, a decrease in ECV causes a decrease in pressure and stretch. Changes in volume sensed by the volume receptors lead to changes in cardiac output, vascular resistance, thirst, and renal handling of sodium and water.

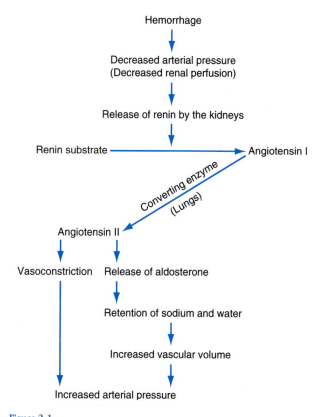

**Figure 2-1**
Action of the renin-angiotensin-aldosterone system: a clinical example.

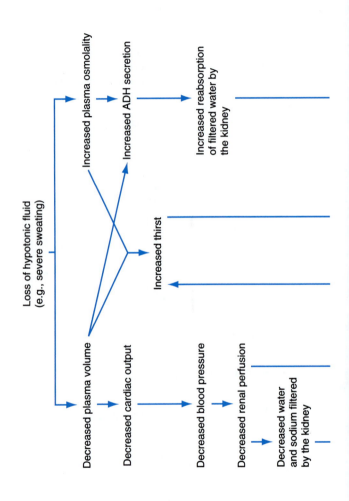

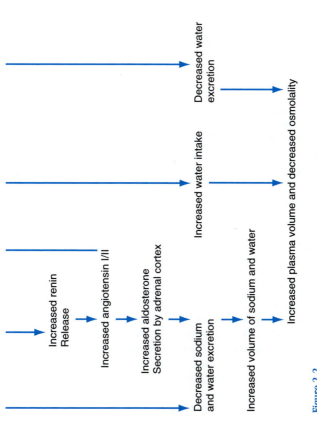

**Figure 2-2**
Regulation of fluid volume and osmolality: a clinical example.

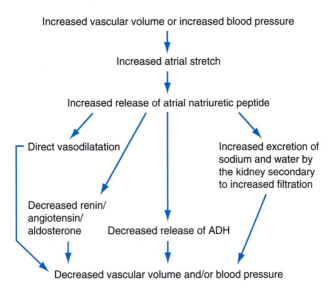

Increased vascular volume or increased blood pressure

↓

Increased atrial stretch

↓

Increased release of atrial natriuretic peptide

Direct vasodilatation

Decreased renin/ angiotensin/ aldosterone

Decreased release of ADH

Increased excretion of sodium and water by the kidney secondary to increased filtration

Decreased vascular volume and/or blood pressure

Figure 2-3
Actions of the atrial natriuretic peptide.

These changes are mediated by a combination of interrelated neurologic and hormonal functions described in subsequent sections.

## Sympathetic Nervous System

The sympathetic nervous system provides the initial compensatory response to rapid or short-term changes in the ECV. Changes in stretch sensed by the volume receptors lead to changes in sympathetic tone. Decreased ECV, for example, results in increased sympathetic tone. Increased sympathetic tone causes the following:

1. **Increased cardiac output:** Secondary to an increase in cardiac contractility, conduction, and rate.
2. **Increased arterial resistance.**
3. **Increased release of renin by the kidneys:** Leads to an increase in the release of aldosterone by the adrenal cortex (see Figure 2-1).

Items 1 and 2 act to raise blood pressure only. Item 3 leads to an increase in both blood pressure and vascular volume, owing to the retention of sodium and water.

## Renin-Angiotensin

Renin is a proteolytic enzyme produced and released by the kidney in response to decreased renal perfusion (secondary to a reduction in ECV) or increased sympathetic nervous system stimulation. Renin acts on angiotensinogen to produce angiotensin I, which is converted to angiotensin II, a potent vasoconstrictor. Angiotensin II, in turn, stimulates the release of aldosterone. Certain antihypertensive medications (e.g., captopril) act in part by preventing the conversion of angiotensin I to angiotensin II.

## Aldosterone

Renin raises blood pressure through the actions of aldosterone. Aldosterone is a mineralcorticoid hormone released by the adrenal cortex, which acts on the distal portion of the renal tubule to increase the reabsorption (saving) of sodium and the secretion and excretion of potassium and hydrogen. Because sodium retention leads to water retention, aldosterone acts as a volume regulator. Factors that increase the release of aldosterone include the following:

1. **Increased renin levels**
2. **Increased plasma potassium levels**
3. **Decreased plasma sodium levels**
4. **Increased adrenocorticotropic hormone levels**

## Atrial Natriuretic Factor

*Atrial natriuretic factor (ANF),* also known as *atrial natriuretic peptide,* is a recently identified hormone released by the cardiac atria in response to increased atrial pressure. In contrast to the renin-angiotensin-aldosterone system, ANF acts to reduce blood pressure and vascular volume. Its actions are believed to include the following:

1. **Increased excretion of sodium and water by the kidney secondary to increased filtration**
2. **Decreased synthesis of renin and decreased release of aldosterone**
3. **Decreased release of antidiuretic hormone (ADH)**
4. **Direct vasodilation**

ANF is released in response to any condition that causes volume expansion, or elevated cardiac filling pressures, e.g., congestive heart failure (CHF), chronic renal failure, use of vasoconstrictor agents, and atrial tachycardia (see Figure 2-3). If analogs (man-made substances with similar structure and function) of ANF can be developed, potentially they may be useful in the management of hypertension, CHF, renal failure, and other volume overload states.

## Antidiuretic Hormone and Thirst

Both ADH and thirst assist in the regulation of vascular volume. For a discussion of their actions see below.

# Regulation of Extracellular Fluid Osmolality

The osmolality or concentration of the ECF determines whether fluid moves into or out of the cells.

*Increased ECF osmolality → cells shrivel*

*Decreased ECF osmolality → cells swell*

Thus it is critical that the ECF osmolality be maintained within a narrow range to protect cellular function. The primary symptoms of altered plasma osmolality are neurologic (e.g., irritability, personality changes, seizures, coma) and reflect the changes in brain cell function.

Because sodium is the primary solute of the ECF, it is also the primary determinant of ECF osmolality. Two control systems work together to maintain the sodium/water ratio: ADH and thirst.

## Antidiuretic hormone

ADH is a produced by the hypothalamus and secreted into the general circulation by the posterior pituitary gland. It acts on the collecting duct in the kidney to increase the reabsorption (saving) of water and allow the excretion of a concentrated urine. Factors that increase the release of ADH are found in the *top* box on p. 21; factors that decrease the release of ADH are found in the *bottom* box on p. 21. ADH is also an arterial vasoconstrictor that acts to raise blood pressure by increasing vascular resistance. ADH is regulated primarily by changes in plasma osmolality and ECV. Additional factors that affect the release of ADH are emotions and medications (see Chapter 20).

In addition to medications that affect the release of ADH, there are also medications that suppress or enhance the action of ADH on the renal collecting duct (see the box on p. 22).

## Factors that Increase the Release of Antidiuretic Hormone (ADH)*

- Increased plasma osmolality sensed by osmoreceptors located within the hypothalamus
- Decreased effective circulating volume sensed by volume receptors located within the pulmonary vasculature and the left atria
- Decreased blood pressure sensed by baroreceptors
- Stress and pain
- Medications, including morphine and barbiturates
- Surgery and certain anesthetics
- Positive pressure ventilators

*See Chapter 20 for a discussion of disorders that lead to inappropriate or excessive production of ADH.

## Factors that Decrease the Release of Antidiuretic Hormone (ADH)*

- Decreased plasma osmolality
- Increased effective circulating volume
- Increased blood pressure
- Medications, including phenytoin and ethyl alcohol

*See Chapter 20 for a discussion of disorders that lead to a reduction in ADH activity or release.

## Thirst

In addition to ADH, thirst also acts to regulate the ECF concentration and is stimulated by essentially the same factors that increase the release of ADH: increased plasma osmolality, volume depletion, and hypotension. Increased angiotensin II levels and dry mucous membranes (the sensation of a dry mouth) also stimulate thirst. Thirst is not as carefully regulated as ADH because it is affected strongly by social and emotional factors. However, thirst does provide the primary protection against hyperosmolality. Symptomatic hyperosmolality occurs only in individuals who do not have a

| Medications that Alter the Action of Antidiuretic Hormone | |
|---|---|
| Suppress | Enhance |
| Lithium | Chlorpropamide |
| Demeclocycline | Indomethacin |
| Methoxyflurane | |

normal thirst mechanism or who do not have access to water. Thus hyperosmolality typically occurs in infants or comatose patients who are unable to ask for water. Alert patients with diabetes insipidus, for example, who excrete a large, abnormally dilute urine because of altered ADH function, will maintain a relatively normal osmolality and volume as long as they are able to drink and satisfy their thirst.

## Defense of Brain Cell Volume

Because the number of particles within most cells remains relatively constant, changes in the osmolality of the fluid surrounding the cells will affect the volume of water within the cells. Thus changes in ECF osmolality affect the volume of the ICF. Although affected by changes in ECF osmolality, especially sudden changes, the brain cells are able to defend against large changes in water volume by varying the number of intracellular particles. This is an important defense, given the critical function and location of the brain. The exact particles involved and the mechanism by which these changes occur remain unclear. Rapid correction of abnormalities in ECF osmolality must be avoided because of the risk of sudden changes in brain cell volume (see Chapter 7).

# Fluid Gains and Losses

3

In health there is a steady state or balance between the fluids gained and lost by the body. As discussed in Chapter 2, the volume, concentration, and composition of body fluids are regulated so that output matches intake and balance is maintained. Loss of hypotonic fluids, for example, leads to decreased water excretion and increased thirst. This physiologic balance is termed *homeostasis*. This chapter reviews the means of normal and abnormal fluid gains and losses. Table 3-1 lists daily fluid gains and losses in approximate amounts.

## Fluid Gains

### Oxidative Metabolism

Approximately 300 ml of water are produced daily by the oxidation of carbohydrates, proteins, and fat. That is, oxygen combines with some of the hydrogen in these substances to produce water. This amount of water is insufficient to compensate for the body's obligatory fluid losses, thus some additional oral, parenteral, or enteral intake is necessary to maintain body volume. Under the best

Table 3-1    Average daily fluid gains and losses in the adult

| Fluid Gains | | Fluid Losses | |
|---|---|---|---|
| Oxidative metabolism | 300 ml | Kidneys | 1200-1500 ml |
| | | Skin | 500-600 ml |
| Oral fluids | 1100-1400 ml | Lungs | 400 ml |
| Solid foods | 800-1000 ml | GI tract | 100-200 ml |
| TOTAL | 2200-2700 ml | TOTAL | 2200-2700 ml |

*GI,* Gastrointestinal.

of conditions, individuals may survive weeks without food intake but only days without water intake.

## Oral Fluids

Approximately 1100 to 1400 ml of fluid are consumed orally per day. Fluid intake varies greatly because thirst is affected by social, emotional, and physiologic factors (see p. 8).

## Solid Food

Fluid is gained through the consumption of solid food, which provides approximately 800 to 1000 ml of water each day. Meat, for example, is approximately 70% water, and fruits and vegetables are over 90% water by weight.

## Fluid Therapy

Fluid also may be gained through parenteral or enteral routes and by means of irrigants that are retained. If a nasogastric (NG) tube is irrigated, for example, and an equal amount is not withdrawn and discarded, the extra irrigant must be considered a fluid gain. Mechanical ventilation with humidified gases may result in a net gain of water by the lungs. See Chapter 6 for a discussion of parenteral fluid therapy and Chapter 26 for a discussion of all types of nutritional therapy.

# Fluid Losses
## Kidneys

The kidneys are the primary regulators of fluid and electrolyte balance. Approximately 180 L of plasma are filtered daily by the kidneys. From this volume, approximately 1500 ml of urine are excreted each day. Hourly urine output has an *average range* of 40 to 80 ml for adults and 0.5 ml/kg/hr for children. The volume, composition, and concentration of urine varies greatly and will depend on intake and other fluid losses. Urine values (volume and concentration) should always be evaluated in relation to the body's need to conserve or excrete fluid. The dehydrated patient who needs to conserve fluid, for example, would be expected to excrete less urine than the patient who is adequately hydrated.

The concentration of urine may range from 50 to 1400 mOsm/kg. Although sodium is the primary determinant of extracellular fluid (ECF) osmolality or concentration, metabolic wastes are the primary determinant of urinary osmolality or concentration. Therefore in severe hypovolemia or hypotension, for example, the kidneys are able to excrete a concentrated yet relatively sodium-free urine.

- **Normal urinary output:** At maximal urinary concentration (1200 mOsm/kg), at least 400 ml of urine must be produced to excrete the daily load of metabolic wastes. Infants, the elderly, and individuals with renal disease who cannot maximally concentrate their urine will have greater obligatory water losses. That is, they will need to produce a proportionately larger volume of urine to excrete their daily load of metabolic wastes. Average daily urine output is 1500 ml in adults.
- **Oliguria:** Urinary output of less than 400 ml in 24 hours. It signals the retention of metabolic wastes.
- **Anuria:** Production of less than 100 ml of urine in 24 hours.
- **Polyuria:** An abnormally large amount of urinary output.

## Skin

An average of 500 to 600 ml of sensible and insensible fluid is lost via the skin each day.

- **Insensible fluid:** Loss is evaporative from the skin and occurs without the individual's awareness. It is lost at a rate of 6 ml/kg/24 hours in the average adult but can increase significantly with fever or burns. Low-birthweight infants, especially those weighing less than 1 kg, are prone to extremely high rates of insensible fluid loss owing to multiple factors, including larger skin surface area and increased skin water content. Use of radiant warmers will significantly increase insensible fluid loss in the neonate. Insensible fluid is nearly electrolyte-free and should be considered pure water loss.
- **Sensible fluid (i.e., sweat):** Important in dissipating body heat, and like insensible fluid, it is hypotonic. Sensible fluid, however, does contain a significant amount of electrolytes (see Table 1-2). The rate of sensible fluid loss varies greatly with the individual's activity level and the ambient temperature. In extreme cases, sensible fluid loss may be as great as 2 L/hr.

# Lungs

Approximately 400 ml of insensible fluid are lost through the lungs each day. This amount may increase with increased respiratory depth or dry climate.

# Gastrointestinal Tract

Under normal conditions, the gastrointestinal (GI) tract accounts for only 100 to 200 ml of fluid loss each day, yet it plays a vital role in fluid regulation because it is the site of nearly all fluid gain. In disease, however, the GI tract may become a site of major fluid loss because approximately 3 to 6 L of isotonic fluid are secreted into and reabsorbed out of the GI tract daily. This is equal to approximately one third of the ECF volume. Thus abnormal GI losses (e.g., NG suction, vomiting, or diarrhea) may lead to profound fluid loss. The composition of the GI secretions varies with the location within the GI tract. Above the pylorus, the losses are isotonic and contain sodium, potassium, chloride, and hydrogen. Below the pylorus, losses are isotonic and contain sodium, potassium, and bicarbonate (see Table 1-2). Diarrhea from the large intestine is hypotonic (see Chapter 18).

# Additional Losses

Significant amounts of fluid may be lost as a result of increased evaporative loss from large open wounds, draining wounds, fistulas, or external bleeding. Crying may contribute significantly to fluid loss in small children.

# Third-Space Losses

The loss of ECF into a normally nonequilibrating space is termed *third-space fluid shift*. Although this fluid is not lost from the body, it is temporarily unavailable for use by either the intracellular fluid or ECF. Third-space fluid losses must be considered when evaluating the adequacy of fluid therapy. See Table 6-1 for a list of disorders associated with third-space fluid shifts.

# Nursing Assessment of the Patient at Risk

## 4

Fluid and electrolyte homeostasis is essential for health and well-being. Unfortunately, fluid, electrolyte, and acid-base disturbances are potential complications of almost all disease states and medical therapies. Nurses in all areas of practice must be diligent in their assessment of individuals at risk for developing fluid, electrolyte, and acid-base disturbances. After an initial assessment and development of diagnoses, ongoing surveillance is critical to ensure adequate treatment or prevention of imbalances.

## Nursing History

Each of the following dimensions of the health history should be considered.

### Physiologic .

1. Does the individual have any disease or disorders that may cause a disturbance in fluid and electrolyte homeostasis (e.g., ulcerative colitis, diabetes mellitus)?
2. Is the individual receiving any medications or therapy that may cause a disturbance in fluid, electrolyte, and acid-base status (e.g., diuretics, nasogastric [NG] suction)?

### Developmental

Is the individual at increased risk because of age or social situation (e.g., an elderly adult who lives alone)? NOTE: Fluid volume deficit is more common in infants and the elderly (see Appendix C).

## Psychologic

Are there behavioral or emotional problems that may increase the risk of fluid, electrolyte, and acid-base disturbances (e.g., denial, noncompliance with a medical regimen in a diabetic teenager)?

## Spiritual

Does the individual have any beliefs, values, or practices that may affect his or her ability to comply with medical interventions (e.g., the Jehovah's Witness with gastrointestinal bleeding who refuses human blood products) or increase the risk for imbalance (e.g., religious fasting)?

## Sociocultural

Are there any social, cultural, financial, or educational factors that place the individual at increased risk or affect his or her ability to comply with medical therapy (e.g., the patient on a fixed income who, in an attempt to save money, fills only the digoxin and diuretic prescriptions but not the potassium supplement prescription)?

# Clinical Assessment

Two of the most important tools for the clinical assessment of fluid balance problems are simple nursing procedures that may be initiated without a physician's order: daily weights and intake and output. Hemodynamic monitoring is an invasive means of assessing fluid balance disorders.

## Daily Weights

Acute weight changes are usually indicative of *acute* fluid changes. Each kilogram of weight lost or gained suggests 1 L of fluid lost or gained. Thus a 2-kg acute weight loss equals a 2-L fluid loss. Weight gains do not necessarily indicate an increase in effective circulating volume but rather an increase in total body volume that may be located in any of the fluid compartments. For accuracy and consistency, weight should be measured at the same time of day, preferably before breakfast. The scale should be balanced before each use, and the individual should be weighed wearing approximately the same clothing. The type of scale (i.e., standing, bed, or chair) should be noted so that whenever possible the same scale can be used.

## Intake and Output

All intake and output (I&O) should be accurately measured whenever possible and all unmeasured volumes estimated and noted. The I&O record should include the following:

1. **Intake:**
   - *Oral fluids:* Ice chips must be included and recorded as fluids at approximately one half their volume. Include all foods that are liquid at room temperature.
   - *Parenteral fluids:* Parenteral fluid containers are often overfilled, and the excess should be discarded during setup or the exact amount given recorded.
   - *Tube feedings:* Often a 30- to 50-ml water flush is given at the end of intermittent tube feedings or periodically during continuous tube feedings. This flush needs to be included in the intake record.
   - *Catheter irrigants:* If the catheter is irrigated or lavaged and an equal amount is not withdrawn and discarded, the extra irrigant should be added to the intake record.

2. **Output:**
   - *Urine output:* Ideally, it is measured hourly.
   - *Liquid feces.*
   - *Vomitus.*
   - *NG drainage.*
   - *Excessive sweating:* May be documented either via a rating system (1+ for noticeable sweating to 4+ for profuse sweating) or by documenting the amount of linen saturated with sweat.
   - *Wound drainage:* May be documented by noting the type and number of dressings saturated, by weighing dressings, or by direct measurement of drainage contained in a gravity or vacuum drainage device (e.g., Hemovac, drainage bags).
   - *Draining fistulas:* If possible, collect drainage in a stoma bag or document amount of dressings or linen saturated.
   - *Rapid or labored respiratory rate:* Will contribute to a patient's insensible fluid loss and should be documented.

## Hemodynamic Monitoring

Hemodynamic monitoring may be useful in evaluating fluid volume abnormalities (Table 4-1).

Table 4-1   Hemodynamic evaluation of fluid volume abnormalities

| Clinical Reading | Potential Cause |
| --- | --- |
| CVP <2 mm Hg or <5 cm $H_2O$ <br> PAP <20/8 mm Hg | Decreased effective circulating volume resulting from true volume depletion (e.g., bleeding), shifting of fluid out of the vascular space (e.g., burns), or vasodilation (e.g., after administration of certain antihypertensive medications) |
| CVP >6 mm Hg or >12 cm $H_2O$ | Fluid overload, poor right ventricular function, or constriction of the pulmonary vascular bed |
| PAP >30/15 mm Hg | Increases in fluid volume or in pulmonary vascular resistance |

*CVP*, Central venous pressure; *PAP*, pulmonary artery pressure.

1. **Central venous pressure (CVP):** Measures mean right atrial pressure and right ventricular end-diastolic pressure by means of a catheter that is inserted in or near the right atrium. A normal reading is 2 to 6 mm Hg or 5 to 12 cm $H_2O$.
2. **Pulmonary artery pressure (PAP):** Measured by means of a catheter passed through the right heart and into the pulmonary artery (PA) with the tip positioned in the pulmonary capillary bed. Normal PAP is 20 to 30/8 to 15 mm Hg. PA diastolic pressures may be used to estimate left ventricular end-diastolic pressure and thus evaluate cardiac performance.

## Vital Signs

The following are examples of changes in vital signs that may signal fluid, electrolyte, or acid-base imbalance.

### Body Temperature

1. **Elevations in body temperature:** May lead to fluid and electrolyte losses as a result of increased insensible loss.

Hypernatremic (elevated sodium) dehydration may cause an elevation in temperature.

2. **Decreases in body temperature:** May result from hypovolemia. In severe fluid volume deficit, the rectal temperature may drop to as low as 35°C (95°F).

## Respiratory Rate and Depth

1. **Increases in respiratory rate and depth:** Increase insensible fluid loss and may contribute to the development of volume depletion.

2. **Rapid, deep respirations:** May be compensation for metabolic acidosis.

3. **Shortness of breath, crackles (rales), or rhonchi:** May signal fluid buildup in the lungs caused by fluid volume excess.

## Heart Rate/Pulses

1. **Heart rate:** Increased heart rate may occur with fluid volume deficit as a compensatory mechanism for maintaining cardiac output.

2. **Bounding pulse:** May signal fluid volume excess. The strength and volume of the pulse is dependent on the volume of blood ejected by the left ventricle and the strength of the left ventricular contraction. Both may increase in fluid volume excess.

3. **Weak, thready pulse:** May signal fluid volume deficit because of a reduction in intravascular volume.

4. **Irregular heart rate:** May occur with hypokalemia or hypomagnesemia secondary to the development of dysrhythmias.

## Blood Pressure

Blood pressure (BP) is determined by multiplying cardiac output (CO) by systemic vascular resistance. CO, in turn, is the product of heart rate multiplied by stroke volume (the amount of blood moved with each contraction of the left ventricle). Thus changes in stroke volume, heart rate, or vascular resistance may result in changes in BP.

1. **Decreased BP:** May signal fluid volume deficit, owing to a reduction in stroke volume. Electrolyte imbalances that cause dysrhythmias may decrease BP if either heart rate or stroke volume is affected.

2. **Elevated BP:** May signal fluid volume excess because of an increase in stroke volume.

# Physical Assessment

The following are some examples of changes noted on physical assessment that may be indicative of fluid, electrolyte, or acid-base imbalance. See individual fluid and electrolyte disorders, Chapters 6 through 11, and the acid-base disorders, Chapters 12 through 17, for additional information.

## Integument

1. **Flushed, dry skin:** May signal fluid volume deficit.
2. **Changes in skin turgor:** May reflect changes in interstitial fluid volume. Turgor may be assessed by pinching skin over the forearm, sternum, or dorsum of the hand. With adequate hydration, the pinched skin returns quickly to its original position when released. With fluid volume deficit, the pinched skin stays elevated for several seconds. This is a less reliable indicator in the elderly, owing to the skin's decreased elasticity. In these individuals, skin turgor is best assessed on the inner aspect of the thigh or over the sternum.
3. **Edema:** Indicates an expanded interstitial volume. It may be localized (usually the result of inflammation) or generalized (because of altered capillary hemodynamics and the retention of excess sodium and water) and usually is most evident in dependent areas. The presence of periorbital edema suggests significant fluid retention. Pitting should be assessed over a bony surface such as the tibia or sacrum and rated according to severity (i.e., 1+ for barely detectable edema to 4+ for deep, persistent pitting [see Figure 6-2]). See Chapter 6 for additional information.
4. **Increased furrowing of the tongue:** Suggestive of fluid volume deficit.
5. **Decreased moisture between the cheek and gum in the oral cavity:** Signals fluid volume deficit.

## Cardiovascular System

1. **Assessment of jugular venous distention:** Provides an estimate of central venous pressure. With the head of bed at a 30- to 45-degree angle, measure the distance between the

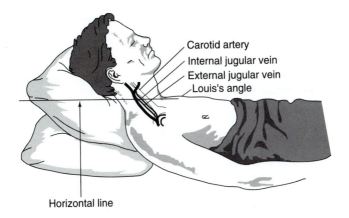

Carotid artery
Internal jugular vein
External jugular vein
Louis's angle

Horizontal line

**Figure 4-1**
Inspection of external jugular venous pressure.
(Redrawn from Thompson J et al: *Clinical nursing,* ed 3, St Louis, 1993, Mosby.)

level of the sternal angle (Louis's angle) and the point at which the internal and external jugular veins collapse. Optimally this distance should be 3 cm or less (Figure 4-1). Values of greater than 3 cm suggest fluid volume excess or decreased cardiac function.

2. **Assessment of the veins of the hands:** May be used to assess fluid volume status. Normally, elevating the hand will collapse the veins in 3 to 5 seconds, and lowering the hand will refill them in 3 to 5 seconds. With fluid volume deficit, the veins of the lowered hand require more than 3 to 5 seconds to fill. With fluid volume excess, the veins of the elevated hand require more than 3 to 5 seconds to empty.

3. **Dysrhythmias:** May occur with potassium, calcium, and magnesium abnormalities (see individual sections for a discussion of specific electrocardiogram changes).

## Neurologic System

1. **Changes in level of consciousness (LOC):** Occur with changes in serum osmolality or changes in serum sodium. The severity of the symptoms depends on the rate and degree

of change. Changes in LOC also may occur with acute acid-base imbalances.

2. **Restlessness and confusion:** May occur with fluid volume deficit or acid-base imbalance.
3. **Abnormal reflexes:** Occur with calcium and magnesium changes. Calcium and magnesium deficits enhance neuro-muscular excitability (e.g., hyperactive reflexes), whereas calcium and magnesium excesses depress neuromuscular function (e.g., diminished reflexes).
4. **Positive Trousseau's sign and Chvostek's sign:** Can occur with hypocalcemia and hypomagnesemia.
   - *Positive Trousseau's sign:* Ischemia-induced carpal spasm. It is elicited by applying a BP cuff to the upper arm and inflating it past systolic BP for 2 minutes.
   - *Positive Chvostek's sign:* Unilateral contraction of the facial and eyelid muscles. It is elicited when irritating the facial nerve by percussing the face just in front of the ear.
5. **Neuromuscular changes resulting from altered membrane polarization of excitable tissue:** Caused by abnormalities in potassium or calcium levels. For example, neuromuscular symptoms of tingling, paresthesias, weakness, and flaccid paralysis may occur with hyperkalemia. Weakness, cramps, dysrhythmias, and paralysis may occur with hypokalemia. Neuromuscular irritability and paresthesias may also occur with metabolic and respiratory alkalosis.

## Gastrointestinal System

1. **Anorexia, nausea, and vomiting:** May occur with acute fluid volume deficit or fluid volume excess.
2. **Thirst:** Symptomatic of increased osmolality or fluid volume deficit.

# Laboratory Assessment of Fluid, Electrolyte, and Acid-Base Balance

Laboratory tests are vital in the early identification and continuous monitoring of fluid, electrolyte, and acid-base imbalances. Consideration of laboratory results should be included in the nursing assessment of patients at risk for fluid, electrolyte, and acid-base disturbances. The laboratory values that follow are applicable to the adult.

## Tests to Evaluate Fluid Status
### Serum Osmolality

*Normal is 280 to 300 mOsm/kg.*
Serum osmolality is the measurement of the number of osmotically active solutes in the serum. It may be measured directly or estimated by doubling the serum sodium because sodium and its accompanying anions are the primary determinants of serum osmolality. A more exact estimate of serum osmolality considers glucose and urea by using the following formula:

$$\text{Serum osmolality} = 2\,Na^+ + \frac{\text{Serum glucose}}{18} + \frac{\text{Urea (BUN)}}{2.8}$$

Because glucose and urea are measured by weight (mg/dl), their values must be converted to concentration (number of particles) by dividing their weight per liter of solution by their molecular weight.

Hence, glucose is divided by 18 and blood urea nitrogen (BUN) is divided by 2.8.

1. **Factors that may increase serum osmolality:**
   - *Free water loss:* For example, insensible water loss (see p. 25 for a discussion of insensible water loss).
   - *Diabetes insipidus:* See Chapter 20 for additional information.
   - *Sodium overload:* For example, excessive administration of sodium bicarbonate ($NaHCO_3$).
   - *Hyperglycemia:* See Chapter 20.
2. **Factors that may decrease serum osmolality:**
   - *Syndrome of inappropriate secretion of antidiuretic hormone (SIADH):* See Chapter 20.
   - *Diuretics.*
   - *Adrenal insufficiency:* See "Addisonian Crisis" in Chapter 20.
   - *Renal failure:* Caused by retention of excess water (see Chapter 22).
   - *Isotonic fluid loss* that is replaced with water or hypotonic fluids, for example, vomiting of isotonic gastric contents with water replacement.

## Hematocrit

*Normals are 40% to 54% (males) and 37% to 47% (females).*
Hematocrit measures the volume (percentage) of whole blood that is comprised of red blood cells (RBCs). Because hematocrit measures the percentage of cells in relation to plasma, it will be affected by changes in plasma volume. Thus the hematocrit will increase with dehydration and decrease with overhydration. The hematocrit may remain normal immediately following an acute hemorrhage (the concentration of RBCs to plasma has not changed), but over a period of hours there is a shift of fluid from the interstitial fluid to the plasma and the hematocrit drops. In addition, the kidneys compensate for the loss of volume by retaining sodium and water.

## Urea Nitrogen

*Normal BUN is 6 to 20 mg/dl.*
Urea is produced by the body as a by-product of hepatic protein metabolism. Its primary means of removal from the body is excretion by the kidneys. Urea production occurs at a fairly steady rate so that increased BUN usually reflects a reduction in renal

function. Urea synthesis and excretion can be affected, however, by such additional factors as hydration, protein intake, and tissue catabolism, thereby limiting the usefulness of BUN as an indicator of renal function.

1. **Factors that may increase BUN:**
   - *Decreased renal function:* If the increase in BUN is solely the result of reduced renal function, the serum creatinine level will increase at approximately the same rate (creatinine to BUN ratio will be 1:10 to 20).
   - *Excessive protein intake.*
   - *Gastrointestinal (GI) bleeding:* Owing to digestion of blood in the gut.
   - *Increased tissue catabolism (breakdown):* For example, with fever, sepsis, or antianabolic steroid use.
   - *Dehydration:* Urea excretion varies with water excretion. In dehydration, decreased water excretion causes decreased urea excretion.

2. **Factors that may decrease BUN:**
   - *Low protein diet.*
   - *Severe liver disease:* Caused by decreased hepatic synthesis.
   - *Volume expansion:* For example, overhydration with intravenous (IV) fluids or pregnancy.

## Urine Osmolality

*Physiologic range is approximately 50 to 1400 mOsm/kg; a typical 24-hour specimen is approximately 300 to 900 mOsm/kg.*

This is a measure of the solute concentration of the urine. Unlike plasma, the primary determinants of urinary osmolality are nitrogenous wastes (e.g., urea, creatinine, uric acid). The kidney is capable of excreting a concentrated, yet almost sodium-free, urine. Although the maximum urine osmolality in the adult may be as high as 1400 mOsm/kg, the neonate is capable of concentrating urine to no greater than 500 mOsm/kg and the child to only 700 mOsm/kg.

NOTE: Urinary values for concentration and composition are normal or abnormal only in relation to what is occurring in the blood. A patient with severe diaphoresis, for example, would be expected to have a relatively high urine osmolality (the kidneys should be compensating for the hypotonic fluid loss by retaining water). In contrast, a patient who has been overhydrated with IV 5% dextrose in water ($D_5W$) would be expected to have a relatively low urine osmolality (the kidneys should be compensating for the excess water intake by excreting a dilute urine). In this case, a relatively high urine osmolality would be abnormal.

1. **Factors that may increase urine osmolality:**
   - *Fluid volume deficit.*
   - *SIADH:* Urine osmolality will be inappropriately high, given the serum osmolality (see Chapter 20).
2. **Factors that may decrease urine osmolality:**
   - *Fluid volume excess.*
   - *Diabetes insipidus:* See Chapter 20 for additional information.

## Urine Specific Gravity

*Physiologic range is 1.001 to 1.040; random specimen with normal fluid intake is approximately 1.010 to 1.020.*

Specific gravity measures the weight of a solution in relation to water (water = 1.000). Urine specific gravity evaluates the kidneys' ability to conserve or excrete water. It is a less reliable indicator of concentration than urine osmolality because specific gravity is affected both by the weight and number of solutes. The presence in the urine of a few large solutes such as glucose or protein may cause a deceptively high specific gravity. Advantages of the test are that it can be performed quickly, easily, and inexpensively at the bedside by nursing staff. Table 5-1 shows the relationship of osmolality to specific gravity.

Factors that increase and decrease specific gravity are the same as those that affect urine osmolality. Some substances that may give a false high specific gravity include glucose, protein, dextran, radiographic contrast material, and medications such as carbenicillin disodium. Children under the age of 2 and elderly adults have a decreased ability to concentrate urine so that the upper limit of specific gravity will be lower in these individuals.

Table 5-1  Relationship of osmolality to specific gravity

| Osmolality | Specific Gravity |
|---|---|
| 350 mOsm/kg | ≈ 1.010 |
| 700 mOsm/kg | ≈ 1.020 |
| 1050 mOsm/kg | ≈ 1.030 |
| 1400 mOsm/kg | ≈ 1.040 (physiologic maximum for urinary concentration) |

# Urine Sodium

*Normal random specimen ranges from 50 to 130 mEq/L.*

Urine sodium levels vary with sodium intake (e.g., increased intake results in increased excretion) and volume status (e.g., sodium is conserved in the presence of a decreased effective circulating volume [ECV]). Levels may be measured from 24-hour specimens or from random specimens.

NOTE: Diuretics and advanced renal failure may increase urine sodium levels.

### Clinical applications of urine sodium levels:

- *Evaluation of volume status.*
- *Differential diagnosis of hyponatremia (decreased serum sodium).*
- *Differential diagnosis of acute renal failure.*

Urine sodium, osmolality, and specific gravity may be helpful in differentiating between oliguria caused by decreased ECV and oliguria secondary to acute tubular necrosis (ATN). In volume depletion or decreased ECV, the kidneys are able to respond appropriately by conserving sodium and concentrating urine. Thus urine sodium will be minimal, urine osmolality will exceed plasma osmolality, and urine specific gravity will be greater than 1.015. In ATN (a type of acute renal failure [see Chapter 22]), the kidneys lose their ability to conserve sodium and concentrate urine appropriately. The urine osmolality will remain fixed at less than 350 mOsm/kg, the specific gravity will be fixed at approximately 1.010, and urine sodium typically will be greater than 20 to 40 mEq/L (Table 5-2).

# Tests to Evaluate Electrolyte Balance

Refer to Chapters 7 through 11 for individual discussions of each of the electrolytes. See Table 5-3 for normal values.

**Table 5-2    Urinary values: hypovolemia vs. acute tubular necrosis**

| Urinary Test | Hypovolemia | Acute Tubular Necrosis |
|---|---|---|
| Urine osmolality (mOsm/kg $H_2O$) | >350 | ≤350 |
| Urine specific gravity | 1.020 | Fixed at ≈ 1.010 |
| Urine sodium | <20 | >40 |

#### Table 5-3    Serum electrolytes: normal ranges

| | |
|---|---|
| Sodium | 135-145 mEq/L |
| Chloride | 95-108 mEq/L |
| Potassium | 3.5-5 mEq/L |
| Total $CO_2$ | 22-28 mEq/L |
| Calcium (total) | 8.5-10.5 mg/dl |
| | 4.3-5.3 mEq/L |
| Magnesium (total) | 1.8-3 mg/dl |
| | 1.5-2.5 mEq/L |
| Phosphorus | 2.5-4.5 mg/dl |
| | 1.7-2.6 mEq/L |

#### Table 5-4    Arterial blood gases: normal ranges

| | |
|---|---|
| pH | 7.35-7.45 |
| $Pa_{CO_2}$ | 35-45 mm Hg |
| $Pa_{O_2}$ | 80-95 mm Hg |
| $O_2$ saturation | 95%-99% |
| $HCO_3^-$ | 22-26 mEq/L |

*Paco₂*, Carbon dioxide tension of arterial blood; *Pao₂*, oxygen tension of arterial blood; *HCO₃⁻*, bicarbonate.

## Tests to Evaluate Acid-Base Balance
## Arterial Blood Gases

Arterial blood gases (ABGs) measure the pH, carbon dioxide ($CO_2$) tension, and oxygen ($O_2$) tension of arterial blood, and $O_2$ saturation of hemoglobin. A bicarbonate level of arterial blood is also included in an ABG test and may be measured directly or calculated from pH and $CO_2$ tension of arterial blood ($Pa_{CO_2}$). ABGs evaluate acid-base balance and pulmonary function. Table 5-4 lists normal ABG values. See Chapter 12 for additional information including a step-by-step guide to ABG analysis.

## Carbon Dioxide Content or Total Carbon Dioxide

*Normal range is 22 to 28 mEq/L.*
Using a venous blood sample, this test measures $CO_2$ content in all its chemical forms: dissolved $CO_2$ ($Pco_2$), bicarbonate ($HCO_3^-$), and carbonic acid ($H_2CO_3$). Carbonic acid exists only briefly, and

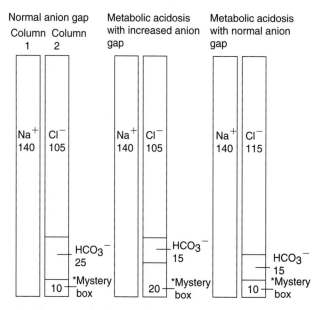

* = Unmeasured anions → Anion gap

Figure 5-1
Anion gap and metabolic acidosis.

therefore its concentration is negligible. Because dissolved $CO_2$ accounts for only 1.2 mEq/L, the $CO_2$ content primarily reflects the bicarbonate level. It will increase in metabolic alkalosis and decrease in metabolic acidosis.

## Anion Gap

*Normal range is 12 ($\pm$2) mEq/L.*
Anion gap reflects the normally unmeasured anions (e.g., phosphates, sulfates, and proteins) in the plasma. Anion gap equals $Na^+ - (Cl^- + HCO_3^-)$. Measurement of the anion gap (Figure 5-1) may be helpful in the differential diagnosis of metabolic acidosis or in identifying hidden metabolic acidosis in certain mixed acid-base disorders (Chapters 15 through 17).

To understand anion gap, think of the extracellular fluid (ECF) as two equal-sized columns—one containing cations (positively charged ions) and the other containing anions (negatively charged ions). Because electroneutrality is maintained at all times within the body, the number of cations and anions (or the size of the two columns as shown in Figure 5-1) must always be equal. Sodium is the body's primary cation, thus the overall size of Column 1 may be determined by measuring serum sodium. The two primary anions of the ECF are chloride and bicarbonate. Their sum ($Cl^-$ mEq/L plus $HCO_3^-$ mEq/L) does not completely fill Column 2. The remaining portion of Column 2 (mystery box) represents the normally unmeasured anions of the ECF. This mystery box (anion gap) may be determined by obtaining a serum electrolyte panel and using the following formula:

Anion gap (mystery box) = $Na^+ - (Cl^- + HCO_3^-)$

The size of the anion gap is significant because the main causes of metabolic acidosis fall into two categories: (1) those that cause an increase in unmeasured anions and thus increase the mystery box/anion gap and (2) those that result from a loss of $HCO_3^-$ or an ingestion or administration of acidifying salts and do not alter the mystery box/anion gap. See the boxes on p. 43 and Chapters 15 and 17 for additional information.

# Urine pH

*Random specimen is 4.6 to 8.*

The kidneys play a critical role in the regulation of acid-base balance by excreting a portion of the hydrogen ions ($H^+$) produced each day. In spite of a buffering system within the renal tubule, which allows maximal excretion of $H^+$ with minimal decrease in urinary pH, the pH of the urine usually is markedly acidic (averaging approximately 6). Measurement of urine pH may be useful in determining if the kidneys are responding appropriately to metabolic acid-base imbalances. Urine pH should decrease in metabolic acidosis and increase in metabolic alkalosis. An inappropriately high urine pH in the presence of metabolic acidosis, for example, suggests renal tubular acidosis (a group of disorders that inhibit renal excretion of $H^+$). An inappropriately low pH in the presence of metabolic alkalosis may signal volume depletion (i.e., sodium bicarbonate is retained as the kidneys attempt to correct the volume deficit by conserving all filtered sodium). Urinary tract infections with pathogens that produce urease cause an alkaline urine because of excess ammonia production. Urine pH should be

## Causes of Metabolic Acidosis with a Normal Anion Gap

### Loss of Bicarbonate

- Diarrhea
- Lower GI fistulas
- Ureterosigmoidostomy
- Renal tubular acidosis
- Early renal insufficiency
- Diuretics: Acetozolamide (Diamox), triamterene (Dyrenium), spironolactone (Aldactone)

### Addition of Acidifying Salts

- Ammonium chloride
- Hyperalimentation fluids without adequate bicarbonate or bicarbonate-producing solutes (e.g., lactate, acetate)
- Lysine hydrochloride
- Arginine hydrochloride

## Causes of Metabolic Acidosis with an Increased Anion Gap

### Retention of Acids

- Renal failure

### Ingestion

- Salicylates
- Methanol
- Paraldehyde

### Abnormal Production of Acids

- Ketoacidosis
- Lactic acidosis

measured within 1 to 2 hours of collection. Urine becomes increasingly alkaline as it sits.

## Lactic Acid

*Normal arterial value is 0.5 to 1.6 mEq/L; venous is 1.5 to 2.2 mEq/L.*

Lactic acid is a by-product of the anaerobic metabolism of glucose. Normally, the small quantity of lactic acid that is produced daily is immediately buffered by $HCO_3^-$, and lactate is generated. This lactate is then converted to $CO_2$ and water or glucose by the liver, and $HCO_3^-$ is regenerated. Any time there is an excess production of lactic acid (e.g., when there is a decreased oxygen delivery to the tissue) or decreased utilization of lactate, dangerous lactic acidosis may develop.

**Factors that may lead to the development of lactic acidosis:**
- *Increased production of lactic acid*
  —Strenuous exercise
  —Shock/sepsis
  —Cardiac arrest
  —Carbon monoxide poisoning
  —Hypoxemia
- *Decreased utilization of lactate*
  —Liver disease
  —Severe acidosis

## Related Tests
## Creatinine

*Normal is 0.6 to 1.5 mg/dl.*

Creatinine is a metabolic waste product produced by the breakdown of muscle creatine. The serum creatinine level reflects the balance between production and excretion by the kidneys. Because it is produced at a steady rate dependent on muscle mass and is not affected by diet, hydration, or tissue catabolism, the creatinine level is a more accurate indicator of renal function than BUN. The serum creatinine level will increase as renal function decreases.

## Serum Albumin

*Normal is 3.5 to 5.5 g/dl.*

Albumin is a small plasma protein produced by the liver that acts osmotically to help hold the intravascular vo lume in the vascular space. Decreased serum albumin (hypoalbuminemia) may lead to the development of edema as a result of the movement of water out of the vascular space and into the interstitial space. The edema seen in protein malnutrition occurs as a result of decreased albumin production.

**Factors that may decrease serum albumin:**

- *Decreased protein intake:* For example, protein malnutrition.
- *Decreased hepatic synthesis:* For example, cirrhosis.
- *Abnormal urinary loss:* For example, nephrotic syndrome.

# DISORDERS OF FLUID, ELECTROLYTE, AND ACID-BASE BALANCE

## II

# Disorders of Fluid Balance

6

## Hypovolemia

Depletion of extracellular fluid (ECF) volume is termed *hypovolemia.* It occurs because of abnormal skin, gastrointestinal (GI), or renal losses; bleeding; decreased intake; or movement of fluid into a nonequilibrating third space (Table 6-1). Depending on the type of fluid lost, hypovolemia may be accompanied by acid-base, osmolar, or electrolyte imbalances. Severe ECF volume depletion can lead to hypovolemic shock. Compensatory mechanisms in hypovolemia include increased sympathetic nervous system stimulation (increased heart rate [HR], inotrophy [cardiac contraction], and vascular resistance), thirst, release of antidiuretic hormone (ADH), and release of aldosterone. Prolonged hypovolemia may lead to the development of acute renal failure (see Chapter 22).

### Assessment

1. **Clinical manifestations:** Dizziness, weakness, fatigue, syncope, anorexia, nausea, vomiting, thirst, confusion, constipation, and oliguria.
2. **Physical assessment:** Decreased blood pressure (BP), especially when standing (orthostatic hypotension); increased HR; poor skin turgor; dry, furrowed tongue; sunken eyeballs; flattened neck veins; increased temperature; and acute weight loss (Table 6-2), except with third spacing. *Infants and children:* Loss of tearing and depressed anterior fontanel.

    The patient in shock will appear pale and diaphoretic with a rapid, thready pulse; they will have supine hypotension, oliguria, and confusion. See the box on p. 51 for assessment changes associated with hypovolemia.
3. **Hemodynamic measurements:** Decreased central venous pressure (CVP), decreased pulmonary artery pressure (PAP),

**Table 6-1 Common disorders associated with third-space* fluid shift**

| Disorder | Pathophysiologic Process |
|---|---|
| Peritonitis | Trapping of fluid and electrolytes in the peritoneal cavity, owing to damage to or inflammation of the peritoneum. As many as 6 liters of fluid can accumulate, depending on degree of acuity. |
| Bowel obstruction | Loss of lower GI fluid caused by sequestering of same in the distended bowel. Several liters may accumulate in the intestinal lumen, leading to a dramatic increase in lumen pressure with eventual damage to intestinal mucosa. |
| Burns | Temporary sequestering of fluid in the interstitial space, owing to increased capillary permeability, decreased vascular colloid osmotic pressure. |
| Ascites | Accumulation of several liters of fluid in the peritoneal cavity, occurring in severe hepatic cirrhosis. Ascites occurs in cirrhosis as a result of hepatic venous obstruction and retention of sodium and water. Symptomatic hypovolemia is most likely to occur after paracentesis because of rapid reaccumulation of ascitic fluid. |
| Fractured hip | Loss of intravascular volume caused by extensive bleeding into the joint. |
| Carcinoma | Trapping of fluid in the interstitial space caused by lymphatic or venous obstruction. |
| Major surgery involving extensive tissue trauma | Abnormal sequestration of fluid at the surgical site because of extensive tissue involvement (e.g., with major abdominal surgery). It also can occur with the loss of ECF into the wall and lumen of the bowel during bowel surgery. |

*There is no third space, per se, but rather, it is a concept describing fluid that is temporarily unavailable either to intracellular fluid or extracellular fluid (ECF). Because third-space fluids are unavailable to the body for its use, the patient exhibits clinical indicators associated with fluid volume deficit, with the exception of weight loss.

Table 6-2    Weight loss as an indicator of extracellular fluid deficit in adults and children

| Acute Weight Loss | Severity of Deficit |
|---|---|
| 2%-5% | Mild |
| 5%-10% | Moderate |
| 10%-15% | Severe |
| 15%-20% | Fatal |

## Assessment Changes with Hypovolemia

| Mild Hypovolemia | Moderate Hypovolemia | Severe Hypovolemia |
|---|---|---|
| Anorexia | Orthostatic | Supine hypotension |
| Fatigue | hypotension | Rapid, thready pulse |
| Weakness | Tachycardia | Cool, clammy skin |
|  | Decreased CVP | Oliguria |
|  | Decreased urine | Confusion, stupor, |
|  | output | coma |

*CVP,* Central venous pressure.

decreased cardiac output (CO), decreased mean arterial pressure (MAP), and increased systemic vascular resistance (SVR).

4. **History and risk factors:**
   - *Abnormal GI losses:* Vomiting, nasogastric (NG) suctioning, diarrhea, and intestinal drainage.
   - *Abnormal skin losses:* Excessive diaphoresis secondary to fever or exercise, burns, and cystic fibrosis.
   - *Abnormal renal losses:* Diuretic therapy, diabetes insipidus, renal disease (polyuric forms), adrenal insufficiency, and osmotic diuresis (e.g., uncontrolled diabetes mellitus, postdye study). See p. 10 for a discussion of osmotic diuresis.
   - *Third spacing or plasma-to-interstitial fluid shift:* Peritonitis, intestinal obstruction, burns, and ascites (see Table 6-1).
   - *Hemorrhage.*
   - *Altered intake:* Coma and fluid deprivation.

## Diagnostic Tests

1. **Blood urea nitrogen (BUN):** May be elevated as a result of dehydration, decreased renal perfusion, or decreased renal function.

2. **Hematocrit:** Elevated with dehydration; decreased in the presence of bleeding. Remember that the hematocrit remains normal immediately following acute hemorrhage, but over a period of hours there is a shift of fluid from the interstitial fluid (ISF) to the plasma and the hematocrit drops (Figure 6-1).

3. **Serum electrolytes:** Variable, depending on type of fluid lost. Hypokalemia often occurs with abnormal GI or renal losses. Hyperkalemia occurs with adrenal insufficiency. Hyper-

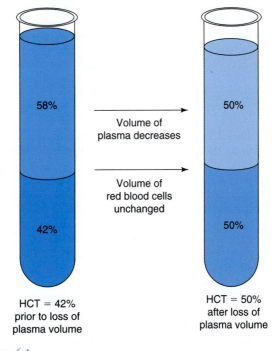

58%

Volume of
plasma decreases

Volume of
red blood cells
unchanged

42%

50%

50%

HCT = 42%
prior to loss of
plasma volume

HCT = 50%
after loss of
plasma volume

**Figure 6-1**
An example of the acute effect of plasma volume loss on hematocrit.

natremia may be seen with increased insensible or sweat losses and diabetes insipidus. Hyponatremia occurs in most types of hypovolemia because of increased thirst and ADH release, which leads to increased water intake and retention, thus diluting the serum sodium. See discussion of individual electrolyte disorders, Chapters 7 through 11.

4. **Serum total carbon dioxide ($CO_2$) ($CO_2$ content):** Decreased with metabolic acidosis and increased with metabolic alkalosis (see "ABG values," below).

5. **Arterial blood gas (ABG) values:** Metabolic acidosis ($pH < 7.35$ and $HCO_3^- < 22$ mEq/L) may occur with lower GI losses, shock, or diabetic ketoacidosis. Metabolic alkalosis ($pH > 7.45$ and $HCO_3^- > 26$ mEq/L) may occur with upper GI losses or diuretic therapy.

6. **Urine specific gravity:** Increased because of the kidneys' attempt to save water; may be fixed at approximately 1.010 in the presence of renal disease; will be decreased in diabetes insipidus.

7. **Urine sodium:** Demonstrates the kidneys' ability to conserve sodium in response to an increased aldosterone level. In the absence of renal disease, osmotic diuresis, diuretic therapy, or hypoaldosteronism, it should be less than 10 to 20 mEq/L.

8. **Serum osmolality:** Variable, depending on the type of fluid lost and the body's ability to compensate with thirst and ADH.

## Collaborative Management

1. **Restoration of normal fluid volume and correction of accompanying acid-base and electrolyte disturbances.** The type of fluid replacement depends on the type of fluid lost and severity of the deficit, serum electrolytes, serum osmolality, and acid-base status.
   **Intravenous fluid therapy.**
   *Crystalloid solutions:*
   - *Dextrose and water:* Provides free water only and will be distributed evenly throughout both intracellular fluid (ICF) and ECF; used to treat total body water deficits only.
   - *Isotonic (normal) saline:* Expands ECF only; does not enter ICF. Usually it is used as an intravascular volume expander or to replace abnormal losses.

■ *Saline/electrolyte solutions:* Provide additional electrolytes (e.g., potassium and calcium) and a buffer (lactate or acetate). Usually hypotonic solutions are used as maintenance fluids, whereas isotonic solutions are used as replacement fluids because most abnormal fluid losses are isotonic.

*Colloid solutions:*

■ *Blood and blood components:* Expand only the intravascular portion of ECF.

■ *Plasma substitutes:* Dextran or hetastarch. Expand the intravascular portion of ECF.

See Tables 6-3 and 6-4 for additional information.

Fluids should be administered rapidly enough and in sufficient quantity to maintain adequate tissue perfusion without overloading the cardiovascular system. The patient's underlying cardiac and renal functions determine how well he or she will tolerate fluid replacement. Thus the rate of fluid administration should be based on both severity of the loss and the individual's hemodynamic response to volume replacement. During a fluid challenge, volumes of fluid are administered at specific rates and intervals, and the patient's hemodynamic response is monitored and documented. Hemodynamic parameters may be prescribed by the physician or, depending on agency policy, determined by a fluid challenge protocol. A typical fluid challenge includes the following steps:

■ Baseline vital signs (VS), hemodynamic measurements (e.g., CVP, PAP, and CO), and clinical data (e.g., breath sounds, skin color and temperature, and sensorium) are obtained.

■ Initial volume of fluid is administered as prescribed or per protocol (e.g., 100 to 200 ml NS over 10 minutes).

■ The patient is reassessed after 10 minutes.

■ If the patient continues to demonstrate signs of hypovolemia (i.e., CVP and PAP remain low), additional fluid may be administered per the physician or agency protocol.

■ If the CVP or PAP increases too rapidly (e.g., >2 mm Hg for the CVP or >3 mm Hg for the PAP), fluid administration is discontinued and the patient is reassessed after 10 minutes. If after 10 minutes the CVP or PAP has dropped and the patient shows no signs of fluid overload, fluid administration is resumed.

■ Fluid administration is continued until the desired hemo-dynamic parameters are achieved or a specific volume has been infused (e.g., 500 to 1000 ml). The fluid challenge should be discontinued if the patient shows signs of fluid volume excess (e.g., crackles [rales], increased HR, increased respiratory rate [RR]), or there is a rapid increase in CVP or PAP.

NOTE: Continued nursing surveillance is essential during and after the fluid challenge.

2. **Restoration of tissue perfusion in hypovolemic shock.** The potential for the development of shock is dependent on both the volume lost (usually >25% of the intravascular volume) and the rapidity of the loss. In turn, successful treatment depends on rapid volume replacement. Initially, hemorrhagic shock is treated with an isotonic electrolyte solution, and packed red blood cells (RBCs) are given as the hematocrit drops. A balanced electrolyte solution (e.g., Ringer's lactate) is recommended because 0.9% NaCl contains excessive amounts of sodium and chloride (see Table 6-3). Fresh frozen plasma is used to replace clotting factors when clotting disorders are present or massive transfusions are necessary. Human albumin, dextran, or hetastarch also may be used to supplement volume replacement (see Table 6-4). Their use, however, remains controversial. Autotransfusion has become an increasingly common therapy in hemorrhagic shock. Autologous blood drained from a sterile body cavity is retransfused within 4 hours of collection via an autotrans-fusion device.

3. **Oral rehydration in pediatric diarrhea:** Oral rehydration solutions have been developed to treat fluid deficit associated with diarrhea, a common source of abnormal fluid loss in infancy and early childhood. These solutions contain varying amounts of glucose, sodium, and potassium and some form of buffer. The glucose concentration of oral rehydration solutions is significant because of the relationship of glucose and sodium reabsorption in the gut. Maximal sodium and water absorption is believed to occur with glucose concen-trations of 10 to 25 g/L. Commonly available fluids, such as cola drinks, ginger ale, and Gatorade, often are prescribed to

*Text continued on p. 65.*

**Table 6-3** Composition and use of commonly prescribed crystalloid solutions

| Solution | Glucose (g/L) | Electrolyte-Composition mEq/L | | | | | Tonicity/mOsm/L | Indications and Considerations* |
|---|---|---|---|---|---|---|---|---|
| | | $Na^+$ | $K^+$ | $Ca^{2+}$ | $Cl^-$ | $HCO_3^-$ | | |
| **Dextrose in Water** | | | | | | | | |
| 1. 5% | 50 | — | — | — | — | — | Isotonic/278 | ■ Provides free water necessary for renal excretion of solutes<br>■ Used to replace water losses and treat hypernatremia<br>■ Provides 170 kcal/L<br>■ Does not provide any electrolytes |
| 2. 10% | 100 | — | — | — | — | — | Hypertonic/556 | ■ Provides free water only, no electrolytes<br>■ Provides 340 kcal/L |
| **Saline** | | | | | | | | |
| 3. 0.45% | — | 77 | — | — | 77 | — | Hypotonic/154 | ■ Provides free water in addition to $Na^+$ and $Cl^-$<br>■ Used to replace hypotonic fluid losses |

| | | | | | | Comments |
|---|---|---|---|---|---|---|
| 4. 0.9% | — | 154 | — | 154 | — | Isotonic/308 | ■ Used as a maintenance solution although it does not replace daily losses of other electrolytes<br>■ Provides no calories |
| 5. 3.0% | — | 513 | — | 513 | — | Hypertonic/1026 | ■ Used to expand intravascular volume and replace ECF losses<br>■ Only solution that may be administered with blood products<br>■ Contains $Na^+$ and $Cl^-$ in excess of plasma levels<br>■ Does not provide free water, calories, or other electrolytes<br>■ May cause intravascular overload or hyperchloremic acidosis<br>■ Used to treat symptomatic hyponatremia |

*Continued*

*Modified from Rose DB: *Clinical pathology of acid-base and electrolyte disorders,* ed 3, New York, 1989, McGraw-Hill Book.
ECF, Extracellular fluid.

**Table 6-3  Composition and use of commonly prescribed crystalloid solutions—cont'd**

| Solution | Glucose (g/L) | Electrolyte-Composition mEq/L | | | | | Tonicity/mOsm/L | Indications and Considerations* |
|---|---|---|---|---|---|---|---|---|
| | | Na$^+$ | K$^+$ | Ca$^{2+}$ | Cl$^-$ | HCO$_3^-$ | | |
| | | | | | | | | ■ Must be administered slowly and with extreme caution because it may cause dangerous intravascular volume overload and pulmonary edema |
| Dextrose in Saline | | | | | | | | |
| 6. 5% in 0.225% | 50 | 38.5 | — | — | 38.5 | — | Isotonic/355 | ■ Provides Na$^+$, Cl$^-$, and free water<br>■ Used to replace hypotonic losses and treat hypernatremia<br>■ Provides 170 kcal/L |
| 7. 5% in 0.45% | 50 | 77 | — | — | 77 | — | Hypertonic/432 | ■ Same as 0.45% NaCl except that it provides 170 kcal/L |
| 8. 5% in 0.9% | 50 | 154 | — | — | 154 | — | Hypertonic/586 | ■ Same as 0.9% NaCl except that it provides 170 kcal/L |

## Multiple Electrolyte Solutions

| | | | | | | | | Comments |
|---|---|---|---|---|---|---|---|---|
| 9. Ringer's | — | 147 | 4 | 5 | 156 | — | Isotonic/309 | ■ Similar in composition to plasma except that it has excess $Cl^-$, no $Mg^{2+}$, and no $HCO_3^-$<br>■ Does not provide free water or calories<br>■ Used to expand the intravascular volume and replace ECF losses |
| 10. Lactated Ringer's (Hartmann's) solution | — | 130 | 4 | 3 | 109 | 28† | Isotonic/274 | ■ Similar in composition to normal plasma except that it does not contain $Mg^{2+}$<br>■ Used to treat losses from burns and lower GI tract<br>■ May be used to treat mild metabolic acidosis but should not be used to treat lactic acidosis<br>■ Does not provide free water or calories |

†In the form of lactate.
*GI,* Gastrointestinal.

**Table 6-4  Composition and use of commonly prescribed colloid solutions**

| Solution | Composition | Volume | Indications and Considerations |
|---|---|---|---|
| **Blood and Blood Components** | | | |
| Whole blood | RBCs, WBCs, platelets, plasma, and some clotting factors | Approximately 500 ml/unit | ■ Used to treat acute massive blood loss, although as most hemorrhagic episodes may be rarely required be treated with packed RBCs and crystalloids<br>■ In the stable patient should increase hematocrit 3% or hemoglobin 1 g/dl/unit<br>■ Requires ABO and Rh compatibility |
| Packed RBCs | RBCs and some plasma ($\approx$ 20%), platelets, and WBCs | 250-350 ml/unit | ■ Administer with 0.9% NaCl only<br>■ Indicated in patients requiring increased $O_2$ carrying capacity, but not necessarily volume expansion<br>■ Less plasma proteins and clotting factors than whole blood<br>■ Requires ABO and Rh compatibility |

| | | | - Specially prepared leukocyte depleted units may be used to decrease the risk of febrile, nonhemolytic transfusion reactions |
|---|---|---|---|
| Fresh frozen plasma | Plasma, plasma proteins, and clotting factors | 200 ml | - Used to restore clotting factors in situations of known deficiency<br>- Although helpful in restoring volume, it should not be used solely for volume expansion<br>- Should be used promptly after thawing to prevent deterioration of clotting factors<br>- Requires ABO compatibility |
| Plasma protein fraction | 5% solution of human plasma proteins (85% albumin, 15% globulins) | 250-500 ml units<br>290 mOsm/L | - Used to expand plasma volume<br>- Greater risk of hypersensitivity reactions than with pure albumin solutions<br>- Does not require typing<br>- Virtually no risk of hepatitis or HIV infection |

RBCs, Red blood cells; WBCs, white blood cells; ABO, blood group system consisting of A, AB, B, and O; Rh, rhesus factor; $O_2$, oxygen; HIV, human immunodeficiency virus.

Continued

Table 6-4    Composition and use of commonly prescribed colloid solutions—cont'd

| Solution | Composition | Volume | Indications and Considerations |
|---|---|---|---|
| Albumin | Human albumin in a buffered saline solution; available in 5% or 25% concentrations | 5% = 250 and 300 ml units 300 mOsm/L<br>25% = 50 and 100 ml units 1500 mOsm/L | ■ Used to expand plasma volume and increase plasma oncotic pressure<br>■ 25% albumin will expand the vascular volume 3 to 4 ml for each ml administered<br>■ Does not require typing<br>■ Virtually no risk of hepatitis or HIV infection<br>■ 25% should be used with caution in persons with cardiac or renal failure because of the risk of intravascular fluid (IVF) overload |

**Plasma Substitutes**

| | | |
|---|---|---|
| Dextran 70 | 6% solution of polysaccharide (average molecular weight of 70,000) combined with saline or dextrose and water | 500 ml/unit |

- Used for rapid volume expansion
- Less expensive than blood products
- May cause bleeding tendencies, interference with crossmatching, and release of histamine

| | | |
|---|---|---|
| Hetastarch | 6% solution of hydroxyethyl starch in saline | 500 ml/unit 310 mOsm/L |

- Used for rapid volume expansion
- Less expensive than blood products
- May cause bleeding tendencies, and circulatory overload
- Should be used with caution in persons with renal failure because of decreased urinary excretion of hetastarch

**Table 6-5** Composition of some oral rehydration solutions

| Formula | $Na^+$ (mEq/L) | $K^+$ (mEq/L) | $Cl^-$ (mEq/L) | Base (mEq/L) | Glucose (g/L) |
|---|---|---|---|---|---|
| Pedialyte (Ross)* | 45 | 20 | 35 | 30 (citrate) | 25 |
| Rehydralyte (Ross) | 75 | 20 | 65 | 30 (citrate) | 25 |
| Infalyte (Mead Johnson) | 50 | 25 | 45 | 34 (citrate) | 30 |
| WHO (World Health Organization)† | 90 | 20 | 80 | 30 (bicarbonate) | 20 |

From Wong D: *Whaley and Wong's nursing care of infants and children*, ed 5, St Louis, 1995, Mosby.
*Note that there are many generic products available with compositions identical to Pedialyte.
†Must be reconstituted with water.

replace fluids lost in mild episodes of diarrhea. However, these are poor choices for fluid replacement in prolonged or severe diarrhea because of their high-glucose and low-electrolyte concentrations. See Table 6-5 for examples of oral rehydration solutions. Commercial oral rehydration solutions are now readily available in pharmacies and markets for home use. However, caregivers must be given explicit instructions concerning the use of oral rehydration solutions. Too-rapid administration may cause gastric distention with reflex vomiting.

4. **Treatment of the underlying cause.**

## Nursing Diagnoses and Interventions

**Fluid volume deficit** related to abnormal loss of body fluids or reduced intake.

**Desired outcomes:** The patient attains adequate intake of fluid and electrolytes as evidenced by urine output of 30 or more milliliters per hour, stable weight, specific gravity 1.010 to 1.030, no clinical evidence of hypovolemia (furrowed tongue, etc.), BP within the patient's normal range, CVP 2 to 6 mm Hg, and HR 60 to 100 beats per minute (bpm). Serum sodium is 135 to 145 mEq/L and hematocrit and BUN are within the patient's normal range. For patients in critical care the following are attained: PAP 20 to 30/8 to 15 mm Hg and CO 4 to 7 L/min.

1. Monitor intake and output (I&O) hourly. Initially, intake should exceed output during therapy. Alert the physician to urine output 30 ml/hr or less for 2 consecutive hours. Measure urine specific gravity every 8 hours. Expect it to decrease with therapy.

2. Monitor VS and hemodynamic pressures for signs of continued hypovolemia. Be alert to decreased BP and CVP and increased HR and SVR. For critical patients, also be alert to decreased PAP, CO, and MAP and to increased SVR.

3. Weigh the patient daily. Daily weights are the single most important indicator of fluid status because acute weight changes are indicative of fluid changes. For example, a 2-kg weight loss equals a 2-L fluid loss. Weigh the patient at the same time of day (preferably before breakfast) on a balanced scale, with the patient wearing approximately the same clothing. Document the type of scale used (i.e., standing, bed, or chair).

4. Administer oral and intravenous (IV) fluids as prescribed. Document response to fluid therapy. Monitor for signs and symptoms of fluid overload or too-rapid fluid administration: crackles, shortness of breath (SOB), tachypnea, tachycardia, increased CVP, increased PAP, neck vein distention, and edema. If the patient is symptomatic of any of the previously mentioned signs and symptoms, follow agency protocol for fluid challenge.

5. Monitor the patient for hidden fluid losses. For example, measure and document abdominal girth or limb size if indicated.

6. Notify the physician of decreases in hematocrit that may signal bleeding. Remember that hematocrit decreases in the dehydrated patient as he or she becomes rehydrated. Decreases in hematocrit associated with rehydration may be accompanied by decreases in serum sodium and BUN.

7. Place the shock patient in a supine position with the legs elevated at 45 degrees to increase venous return. This position returns approximately 500 ml of blood pooled in the veins of the legs to the central circulation. Avoid the Trendelenburg position because this causes abdominal viscera to press on the diaphragm, thereby impairing ventilation. If shock occurs secondary to hemorrhage, draw blood for possible type and crossmatch and ensure that the patient has a No. 16- to 18-gauge IV access to allow rapid administration of packed red blood cells. Insert a Foley catheter to monitor hourly urine output because hourly output reflects the adequacy of fluid replacement.

8. Securely tape all nonLuer-Lok connections on IV lines to prevent bleeding caused by accidental disconnection. Luer-Lok-type connections *must* be used on arterial lines because of the high risk of hemorrhage and on central lines because of the additional risk of air embolus.

**Altered cerebral, renal, and peripheral tissue perfusion** related to hypovolemia.

**Desired outcomes:** The patient has adequate perfusion as evidenced by alertness, warm and dry skin, BP within the patient's normal range, HR less than 100 bpm, urinary output of 30 or more milliliters per hour for 2 consecutive hours, capillary refill less than 2 seconds, and peripheral pulses greater than 2+ on a 0 to 4+ scale.

1. Monitor for signs of decreased cerebral perfusion: vertigo, syncope, confusion, restlessness, anxiety, agitation, excitability, weakness, nausea, and cool and clammy skin. Alert the physician to worsening symptoms. Document response to fluid therapy.

2. Protect patients who are confused, dizzy, or weak. Keep side rails up and bed in lowest position, with wheels locked. Assist with ambulation in step-down units. Raise the patient to sitting or standing positions slowly. Monitor for indicators of orthostatic hypotension: decreased BP, increased HR, dizziness, and diaphoresis. If symptoms occur, return the patient to supine position.

3. To avoid unnecessary vasodilation, treat fevers promptly.

4. Reassure the patient and significant others that sensorium changes will improve with therapy.

5. Monitor I&O and alert the physician to urine output less than 30 ml/hr for 2 consecutive hours. Prolonged reduction in renal perfusion may result in ischemic damage to the kidneys and acute renal failure.

6. Evaluate capillary refill, noting whether it is brisk (<2 seconds) or delayed (≥2 seconds). Notify the physician if refill is delayed.

7. Palpate peripheral pulses bilaterally in the arms and legs (radial, brachial, dorsalis pedis, and posterior tibial). Use a Doppler if unable to palpate pulses. Rate pulses on a 0 to 4+ scale. Notify the physician if pulses are absent or barely palpable. NOTE: Abnormal pulses also may be caused by a local vascular disorder.

For additional nursing diagnoses, see specific medical disorder, electrolyte imbalance, or acid-base disturbance.

## Patient-Family Teaching Guidelines

Give the patient and significant others verbal and written instructions for the following:

1. Signs and symptoms of hypovolemia.

2. Importance of maintaining adequate intake, especially in small children and the elderly, who are more likely to develop dehydration.

3. Medications: name, purpose, dosage, frequency, precautions, and potential side effects.

# Hypervolemia

Expansion of ECF volume is termed *hypervolemia.* It occurs whenever there is (1) chronic stimulus to the kidney to save sodium and water; (2) abnormal renal function, with reduced excretion of sodium and water; (3) excessive administration of IV fluids; or (4) interstitial-to-plasma fluid shift. Hypervolemia can lead to heart failure and pulmonary edema (see Chapter 21), especially in the patient with cardiovascular dysfunction. Compensatory mechanisms for hypervolemia include the release of atrial natriuretic peptide (ANP [see Chapter 2]), leading to increased filtration and excretion of sodium and water by the kidneys and decreased release of aldosterone and ADH. Abnormalities in electrolyte homeostasis, acid-base balance, and osmolality often accompany hypervolemia.

## Assessment

1. **Clinical manifestations:** SOB and orthopnea.
2. **Physical assessment:** Edema, weight gain, increased BP (decreased BP as the heart fails), bounding pulses, ascites, crackles (rales), rhonchi, wheezes, tachypnea, distended neck veins, moist skin, tachycardia, and gallop rhythm.
3. **Hemodynamic measurements:** Increased CVP, PAP, and MAP.
4. **History and risk factors**
   - *Retention of sodium and water:* Heart failure, cirrhosis, nephrotic syndrome, and excessive administration of glucocorticosteroids.
   - *Abnormal renal function:* Acute or chronic renal failure with oliguria.
   - *Excessive administration of IV fluids.*
   - *Interstitial-to-plasma fluid shift:* Remobilization of fluid after treatment of burns, excessive administration of hypertonic solutions (e.g., mannitol, hypertonic saline), or colloid oncotic solutions (e.g., albumin).

## Diagnostic Tests

Laboratory findings are variable and usually nonspecific.

1. **Hematocrit:** Decreased because of hemodilution.
2. **BUN:** Increased in renal failure.
3. **ABG values:** May reveal hypoxemia (decreased $Pao_2$) and

respiratory alkalosis (increased pH and decreased $Paco_2$) in the presence of pulmonary edema.

4. **Serum sodium and serum osmolality:** Decreased if hypervolemia occurs as a result of excessive retention of water (e.g., in chronic renal failure).

5. **Urinary sodium:** Elevated if the kidney is attempting to excrete excess sodium. Urinary sodium will not be elevated in conditions with secondary hyperaldosteronism (e.g., congestive heart failure, cirrhosis, nephrotic syndrome) because hypervolemia occurs secondary to a chronic stimulus to the release of aldosterone.

6. **Urine specific gravity:** Decreased if the kidney is attempting to excrete excess volume. May be fixed at 1.010 in acute renal failure.

7. **Chest x-ray:** May reveal signs of pulmonary vascular congestion.

## Collaborative Management

The goal of therapy is to treat the precipitating problem and return ECF to normal. Treatment may include the following:

1. **Restriction of sodium and water:** See the box below for a list of foods high in sodium.

2. **Diuretics.**

3. **Dialysis or continuous arteriovenous hemofiltration:** In renal failure or life-threatening fluid overload.

NOTE: Also see specific discussions on acute renal failure, Chapter 22, and burns, Chapter 25.

### Foods that are High in Sodium Content

| | |
|---|---|
| Bouillon | Olives |
| Celery | Pickles |
| Cheeses | Preserved meat |
| Dried fruits | Salad dressings and prepared |
| Frozen, canned, or | sauces |
| packaged foods | Sauerkraut |
| Monosodium glutamate | Snack foods (e.g., crackers, |
| (MSG) | chips, pretzels) |
| Mustard | Soy sauce |

**ndx:** Nursing Diagnoses and Interventions

**Fluid volume excess** related to excessive fluid or sodium intake or compromised regulatory mechanism.

**Desired outcomes:** The patient is normovolemic as evidenced by adequate urinary output of at least 30 to 60 ml/hr, specific gravity of approximately 1.010 to 1.020, stable weights, and absence of edema. BP is within the patient's normal range, CVP is 2 to 6 mm Hg, and HR is 60 to 100 bpm. In addition, for critical care patients PAP is 20 to 30/8 to 15 mm Hg, MAP is 70 to 105 mm Hg, and CO is 4 to 7 L/min.

1. Monitor I&O hourly. With the exception of oliguric renal failure, urine output should be more than 30 to 60 ml/hr. Measure urine specific gravity every shift. If the patient is diuresing, specific gravity should be below 1.010 to 1.020.

2. Observe for and document presence of edema: pretibial, sacral, periorbital. Rate pitting on a 1 to 4 scale (Figure 6-2).

3. Weigh the patient daily. Daily weights are the single most important indicator of fluid status. For example, a 2-kg acute weight gain is indicative of a 2-L fluid gain. Weigh the patient at the same time each day (preferably before breakfast) on a balanced scale, with the patient wearing approximately the same clothing. Document the type of scale used (i.e., standing, bed, or chair).

4. Obtain an accurate dietary history and limit sodium intake as prescribed by the physician (see the box on p. 69). Consider use of salt substitutes. NOTE: Salt substitutes contain

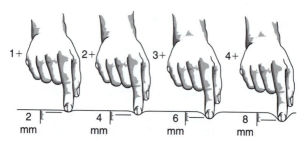

Figure 6-2
Assessment of pitting edema: 1+; 2+; 3+; 4+.

potassium and may be contraindicated in patients with renal failure or in patients receiving potassium-sparing diuretics (e.g., spironolactone, triamterene). Incorporate cultural considerations when providing dietary counseling.

5. Limit fluids as prescribed. Offer a portion of allotted fluids as ice chips to minimize the patient's thirst. Teach the patient and significant others the importance of fluid restriction and how to measure fluid volume.

6. Provide oral hygiene at frequent intervals to keep oral mucous membrane moist and intact.

7. Document response to diuretic therapy. Many diuretics (e.g., furosemide, thiazides) cause hypokalemia. Observe for indicators of hypokalemia: muscle weakness, dysrhythmias (especially premature ventricular contractions [PVCs] and electrocardiogram [ECG] changes—flattened T wave, presence of U waves) (see p. 97). Potassium-sparing diuretics (e.g., spironolactone, triamterene) may cause hyperkalemia: weakness, ECG changes (e.g., peaked T wave, prolonged PR interval, widened QRS) (see p. 103). Notify the physician of significant findings.

8. Observe for physical indicators of overcorrection and dangerous volume depletion secondary to therapy: vertigo, weakness, syncope, thirst, confusion, poor skin turgor, flat neck veins, acute weight loss. Monitor VS and hemodynamic parameters for signs of volume depletion occurring with therapy: decreased BP, CVP, PAP, MAP, and CO; increased HR. Alert the physician to significant changes or findings.

**Impaired gas exchange** related to alveolar-capillary membrane changes secondary to pulmonary vascular congestion occurring with ECF expansion.

**Desired outcomes:** The patient has adequate gas exchange as evidenced by a RR of 20 or fewer breaths per minute, HR 100 or fewer breaths per minute, and $Pao_2$ 80 mm Hg or higher. The patient does not exhibit crackles, gallops, or other clinical indicators of pulmonary edema. For patients in critical care, PAP is less than or equal to 30/15 mm Hg.

1. Acute pulmonary edema is a potentially life-threatening complication of hypervolemia. Monitor the patient for indicators of pulmonary edema, including air hunger, anxiety, cough with production of frothy sputum, crackles (rales),

rhonchi, tachypnea, tachycardia, gallop rhythm, and elevation of PAP and pulmonary artery wedge pressure (PAWP).

2. Monitor ABGs for evidence of hypoxemia (decreased $Pao_2$) and respiratory alkalosis (increased pH and decreased $Paco_2$) or pulse oximetry for decreased oxygen saturation. Increased oxygen requirements are indicative of increasing pulmonary vascular congestion.

3. Keep the patient in semi-Fowler's position or in a position of comfort to minimize dyspnea. Avoid restrictive clothing.

4. Administer oxygen ($O_2$) according to unit protocol or the physician's prescription.

**Impaired tissue integrity** related to edema secondary to fluid volume excess.

**Desired outcome:** The patient's skin remains free of erythema, sores, and ulcerations.

1. Assess and document circulation to extremities at least every shift. Note color, temperature, capillary refill, and peripheral pulses. Determine whether capillary refill is brisk (<2 seconds) or delayed (≥2 seconds). Palpate peripheral pulses bilaterally in the arms and legs (radial, brachial, dorsalis pedis, and posterior tibial). Use Doppler if unable to palpate pulses. Notify the physician if capillary refill is delayed or pulses are absent.

2. Turn and reposition the patient at least every 2 hours to minimize tissue pressure.

3. Check tissue areas at risk with each position change (e.g., heels, sacrum, and other areas over bony prominences).

4. Use special air or fluidized mattress to minimize pressure.

5. Support the arms and hands on pillows and elevate the legs to decrease dependent edema (unless pulmonary edema or heart failure is present).

6. Treat decubitus ulcers with occlusive dressings (e.g., Duoderm, Op-Site, Tegaderm) as per unit protocol. Notify the physician of the presence of sores, ulcers, or areas of tissue breakdown in patients who are at increased risk for infection (e.g., diabetics, immunosuppressed individuals, those with renal failure).

 ## Patient-Family Teaching Guidelines

Give the patient and significant others verbal and written instructions for the following:

1. Signs and symptoms of hypervolemia.
2. Symptoms that necessitate physician notification after hospital discharge: SOB, chest pain, and new pulse irregularity.
3. Low sodium diet, if prescribed; use of salt substitute; avoiding foods that are high in sodium (see the box on p. 69); and high potassium diet or need for potassium supplement if on loop or thiazide-type diuretics. (See the box on p. 100.)
4. Medications, including name, purpose, dosage, frequency, precautions, and potential side effects; signs and symptoms of hypokalemia if the patient is taking diuretics.
5. Importance of fluid restriction if hypervolemia continues.
6. Importance of daily weights.
7. Take once-daily doses of diuretics in the morning to minimize night voiding. If taking twice a day, take the second dose no later than 4 PM.
8. If on diuretics, avoid prolonged standing and rise slowly from lying or sitting to prevent postural hypotension.

## Edema Formation

Edema occurs as a result of expansion of the ISF volume and is defined as a palpable swelling of the interstitial space that is either localized (e.g., thrombophlebitis with venous obstruction) or generalized (e.g., cardiac failure). Severe generalized edema is termed *anasarca*. Edema may develop any time there is an alteration in capillary hemodynamics favoring either increased formation or decreased removal of ISF (Figure 6-3). Increased capillary hydrostatic pressure from volume expansion or venous obstruction, or increased capillary permeability, owing to burns, allergy, or infection, causes an increase in interstitial fluid volume. Decreased removal of ISF occurs when there is an obstruction to lymphatic outflow or a decrease in plasma oncotic pressure (remember that the plasma proteins help hold the vascular volume in the vascular space). Furthermore, retention of sodium and water by the kidneys enhances and maintains generalized edema. This may result from a decreased ability to excrete sodium and water (overflow) as in renal failure, or an increased stimulus to conserve sodium and water (underfilling). In heart failure, for example, impaired cardiac function leads to a reduction in CO with a drop in extracellular volume, which in turn stimulates the kidneys to

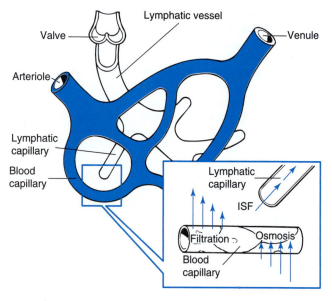

Figure 6-3
Capillary diagram.

conserve sodium and water via the renin-angiotensin system. As the patient with heart failure retains volume, the venous circuit expands, capillary hydrostatic pressure increases, and edema is formed. The edema seen in nephrotic syndrome and hepatic cirrhosis (ascites [see Chapter 24]) is the result of both underfilling and overflow.

## Assessment

Generalized edema usually is most evident in dependent areas. The ambulatory patient exhibits pretibial or ankle edema, whereas the patient restricted to bed exhibits sacral edema. Generalized edema also may present around the eyes (periorbital) or in the scrotal sac because of the low tissue pressures in these areas. Sacral edema may be identified by pressing the index finger firmly into the sacral tissue and maintaining the pressure for several seconds. If a pit remains after the finger has been withdrawn, edema is present. Pitting also may be assessed over the tibia or ankle. Pitting should be rated according to severity (see Figure 6-2). See Chapter 21 for a discussion of pulmonary edema.

## Collaborative Management

1. **Treatment of the primary problem:** For example, digitalis for patients with congestive heart failure.
2. **Mobilization of edema:** For example, with bed rest and supportive hose.
3. **Dietary restrictions of sodium and fluids:** In addition, hidden sodium sources (e.g., medications) should be avoided.
4. **Diuretic therapy:** See below.
5. **Dialysis or continuous arteriovenous hemofiltration:** In renal failure or life-threatening fluid overload.
6. **Abdominal paracentesis:** For the treatment of severe ascites that adversely affects cardiopulmonary functioning.

## Diuretic Therapy

Diuretics reduce edema by inhibiting the reabsorption of sodium and water by the kidneys. Diuretics also may induce the loss of other important electrolytes and alter acid-base balance. Although retention of sodium and water by the kidneys is an important component in the development of edema, not all edematous states require treatment with diuretics. Reduction in the effective circulating volume and alterations in electrolyte balance caused by diuretics may be detrimental. Patients with hepatic cirrhosis, for example, may develop hepatic coma or hepatorenal syndrome with overuse of diuretics, related to diuretic-induced hypokalemia, metabolic alkalosis, and rapid fluid removal. The majority of edematous patients, however, may benefit by the judicious use of diuretics.

The quantity and characteristics of the diuresis varies, depending on the type of diuretic and its site of action within the renal tubule (Figure 6-4 and Table 6-6). Although there are some complications of diuretic therapy that are common to all or most diuretics (see discussion below), the specifics of nursing care will depend on the type of diuretic the patient is receiving (see Table 6-6).

## Complications of Diuretic Therapy

1. **Volume abnormalities:** Volume depletion caused by over-diuresis. Monitor patients for signs of fluid volume deficit: dizziness, weakness, fatigue, and postural hypotension.

Table 6-6  Diuretic action

| Diuretic (by Primary Site of Action) | Potency | Characteristic of Diuresis |
|---|---|---|
| **Proximal Tubule** | | |
| Acetazolamide (Diamox)* | Weak | $NaHCO_3$ diuresis with the loss of additional $Na^+$, $Cl^-$, and $K^+$ |
| **Proximal Tubule and Loop** | | |
| Mannitol† | Moderate | Osmotic diuresis with the loss of water in excess of $Na^+$ and $Cl^-$ |
| **Loop of Henle** | | |
| Furosemide (Lasix)‡ | Strong | Large diuresis (may affect 25% of filtered load of sodium) with loss of $Na^+$, $Cl^-$, and $K^+$ |
| Ethacrynic acid (Edecrin)‡ | Strong | Same as above |
| Bumetanide (Bumex) | Strong | Same as above |
| Torsemide (Demadex)‡ | Strong | Same as above |
| **Early Distal Tubule** | | |
| Thiazides (Diuril, Hydrodiuril, Esidrix)§ | Moderate | Diuresis affecting up to 5% of filtered load of sodium, with loss of $Cl^-$ and $K^+$ |
| Metolazine (Zaroxolyn)§ | Similar to thiazides | |
| Chlorthalidone (Hygrotin)§ | Similar to thiazides | |

| Late Distal Tubule—Potassium-sparing diuretics | | |
|---|---|---|
| Spironolactone (Aldactone)‖ | Weak | Blocks the action of aldosterone, with loss of $Na^+$ and $Cl^-$ but not $K^+$ |
| Triamterene (Dyrenium)‖ | Weak | Weak diuresis with loss of $Na^+$ and $Cl^-$ but not $K^+$; does not depend on the presence of aldosterone |
| Amiloride (Midamor)‖ | Weak | Same as above |

**Clinical indications and nursing considerations:**

*May be used in the treatment of metabolic alkalosis or in combination with other diuretics to treat refractory edema. It is most commonly used to treat glaucoma because it decreases the formation of aqueous humor. It is contraindicated in patients with acidosis. Monitor patients for hypokalemia (see Chapter 8).

†May cause hyperosmolality and circulatory overload owing to the osmotic shift of fluid out of the cells and into the interstitium and intravascular space. Use with caution in patients with decreased cardiac function. Monitor for signs of circulatory overload (e.g., crackles, shortness of breath, tachycardia). It may be used in the treatment of early acute renal failure.

‡Used to treat edema of congestive heart failure and advanced renal failure. It may be used alone or in combination with mannitol or dopamine to reverse early acute renal failure. It is effective in the treatment of acute pulmonary edema owing to its diuretic and direct venous vasodilatory actions. Do not give intravenously rapidly because of the risk of ototoxicity (tinnitus or hearing loss). Stop the infusion and notify the physician if the patient complains of ringing in the ears. Monitor for hypokalemia (see Chapter 8) and volume depletion (see this chapter).

§Often used to treat hypertension owing to diuretic action and antihypertensive effect, which is unrelated to diuretic action. This group of diuretics has the most nondiuresis-related side effects (e.g., decreased release of insulin, hyperlipidemia, skin rashes). Monitor patient for hypokalemia (see Chapter 8), hyperglycemia, and volume depletion (see this chapter). These diuretics also may cause hyperuricemia and hypercalcemia (see Chapter 9).

‖May be combined with the thiazide diuretics for increased diuretic action and less hypokalemia. These diuretics may cause hyperkalemia (see Chapter 8). Avoid concurrent use of other potassium-sparing diuretics or use of salt substitutes.

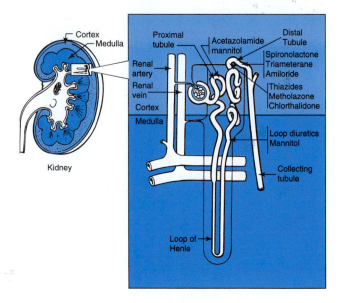

Cortex
Medulla

Proximal
tubule

Acetazolamide
mannitol

Distal
Tubule

Spironolactone
Triameterane
Amiloride

Renal
artery

Renal
vein

Cortex

Medulla

Thiazides
Metholazone
Chlorthalidone

Loop diuretics
Mannitol

Collecting
tubule

Kidney

Loop of
Henle

Figure 6-4
Sites of diuretic action.

2. **Electrolyte disturbances:**

   ■ *Hypokalemia:* Occurs as a result of increased secretion and excretion of potassium by the kidneys. It may occur with all the diuretics except for those that work in the late distal tubule. Hypokalemia can be avoided by giving a potassium-sparing diuretic (see Table 6-6) or a potassium supplement. Monitor patients for indicators of hypokalemia (e.g., fatigue, muscle weakness, leg cramps, irregular pulse).

   ■ *Hyperkalemia:* Occurs because of decreased secretion and excretion of potassium by the kidneys. It may occur with diuretics that work in the late distal tubule (see Table 6-6). The potassium-sparing diuretics should not be given to patients with decreased renal function (because of the increased risk of hyperkalemia) or to patients receiving a

potassium supplement. Monitor patients for indicators of
hyperkalemia: irritability, anxiety, abdominal cramping,
muscle weakness (especially in the lower extremities), and
ECG changes (see Chapter 8 for additional information).

■ *Hyponatremia:* Occurs because of an increased stimulus to
the release of ADH secondary to a reduction in effective
circulating volume (remember that ADH affects the
reabsorption and retention of water only). It is most
common with the thiazide-type diuretics. Monitor patients
for indicators of hyponatremia: irritability, apprehension,
and dizziness.

■ *Hypomagnesemia:* Occurs because of decreased reabsorption and increased excretion of magnesium by the kidneys.
This may occur with the loop and thiazide-type diuretics
and contributes to the development of hypokalemia.
Monitor patients for indicators of hypomagnesemia:
confusion, cramps, and dysrhythmias. Unfortunately, most
magnesium loss occurs from the intracellular space, and
serum values may remain deceptively normal.

3. **Acid-base disturbances:**

■ *Metabolic alkalosis:* May be caused by the loop and
thiazide-type diuretics because of an increased secretion
and excretion of hydrogen by the kidneys and the
contraction of the ECF around the existing bicarbonate
(contraction alkalosis). Monitor patients for indicators of
metabolic alkalosis: muscular weakness, dysrhythmias,
apathy, and confusion.

■ *Metabolic acidosis:* May occur as a result of increased loss
of bicarbonate in the urine with acetazolamide. Monitor
patients for indicators of metabolic acidosis: tachypnea,
fatigue, and confusion. Metabolic acidosis also may occur
with the potassium-sparing diuretics.

4. **Other metabolic complications:**

■ *Azotemia:* This is increased retention of metabolic wastes
(e.g., urea and creatinine) resulting from a reduction in
effective circulating volume with decreased perfusion of
the kidneys and decreased excretion of metabolic wastes.
Alert the physician to changes in BUN and serum
creatinine levels.

■ *Hyperuricemia:* Occurs as a result of increased reabsorption and decreased excretion of uric acid by the kidneys.

Alert the physician to patient complaints of gouty type pain. This condition usually is problematic only in patients with preexisting gout.

## Intravenous Fluid Therapy

The goals of IV fluid therapy are to maintain or restore normal fluid volume and electrolyte balance and to provide a means of administering medications quickly and efficiently. An additional concern is that of nutrition. Unfortunately, routine IV fluids (i.e., 5% dextrose solutions) contain only enough carbohydrates to minimize tissue breakdown and starvation. They do not provide adequate calories and essential amino acids needed for tissue synthesis. For example, 5% dextrose solutions supply only 170 to 200 calories per liter, whereas the average patient on bed rest

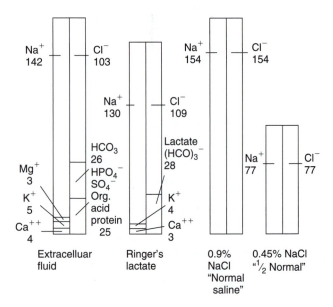

**Figure 6-5**
Comparison of extracellular fluid and three common intravenous solutions (29 mEq/L).

requires a minimum of 1500 calories a day. Patients should not be maintained solely on 5% dextrose solutions for longer than a few days. See Chapter 26 for a discussion of nutritional therapies and total parenteral nutrition (TPN).

The type of IV fluid prescribed for volume replacement or maintenance depends on several factors, including the type of fluid lost and the patient's nutritional needs, serum electrolytes, serum osmolality, and acid-base balance. See Figure 6-5 for a comparison of lactated Ringer's solution, 0.9% NaCl, and 0.45% NaCl to ECF.

## Commonly Prescribed Intravenous Fluids

IV fluids are divided into two major categories: crystalloids and colloids. *Crystalloid solutions* contain only electrolytes and glucose, substances that are not restricted to the intravascular space. Therefore these solutions will expand the entire extracellular space. Depending on their sodium content, crystalloids also may expand the ICF volume. Isotonic NaCl (0.9%) expands only the ECF, whereas hypotonic NaCl solutions and dextrose and water solutions

*Text continued on p. 86.*

### When a Transfusion Reaction Occurs

1. STOP THE TRANSFUSION.
2. Keep the intravenous line open with 0.9% normal saline.
3. Report the reaction to both the transfusion service and attending physician immediately.
4. Do a clerical check at bedside of identifying tags and numbers.
5. Treat symptoms per physician's order and monitor vital signs.
6. Send the blood bag with the attached administration set and labels to the transfusion service.
7. Collect blood and urine samples and send them to the laboratory.*
8. Document thoroughly on a transfusion reaction form and in the patient's chart.

From National Blood Resource Education Programs, Transfusion therapy guidelines for nurses, September, 1990, NIH Publication No. 90-2668a.
*Check with the transfusion service to determine the specific blood and urine samples needed to evaluate reactions.

Table 6-7  Acute transfusion reactions

| Reaction | Cause | Clinical Manifestations | Management | Prevention |
|---|---|---|---|---|
| Acute hemolytic | Infusion of ABO-incompatible whole blood, RBCs, or components containing 10 ml or more of RBCs. Antibodies in the recipient's plasma attach to antigens on transfused RBCs causing RBC destruction. | Chills, fever, low back pain, flushing, tachycardia, tachypnea, hypotension, vascular collapse, hemoglobinuria, hemoglobinemia, bleeding, acute renal failure, shock, cardiac arrest, death. | Treat shock, if present. Draw blood samples for serologic testing slowly to avoid hemolysis from the procedure. Send urine specimen to the laboratory. Maintain BP with IV colloid solutions. Give diuretics as prescribed to maintain urine flow. Insert indwelling catheter or measure voided amounts to monitor hourly urine output. Dialysis may be required | Meticulously verify and document patient identification from sample collection to component infusion. |

| | | | | if renal failure occurs. Do not transfuse additional RBC-containing components until transfusion service has provided newly crossmatched units. | |
| Febrile, non-hemolytic (most common) | Sensitization to donor white blood cells, platelets or plasma proteins. | Sudden chills and fever (rise in temperature of greater than 1°C), headache, flushing, anxiety, muscle pain. | Give antipyretics as prescribed—avoid aspirin in thrombocytopenic patients. **Do not restart transfusion.** | Consider leukocyte-poor blood products (filtered, washed, or frozen). |
| Mild allergic | Sensitivity to foreign plasma proteins. | Flushing, itching, urticaria (hives). | Give antihistamine as directed. If symptoms are mild and transient, transfusion may be restarted slowly. | Treat prophylactically with antihistamines. |

From National Blood Resource Education Programs: *Transfusion therapy guidelines for nurses*, September, 1990, NIH Publication No. 90-2668a.
*ABO*, Blood group consisting of groups A, AB, B, and O; *RBCs*, red blood cells; *BP*, blood pressure; *IV*, intravenous.                                    *Continued*

**Table 6-7**  Acute transfusion reactions—cont'd

| Reaction | Cause | Clinical Manifestations | Management | Prevention |
|---|---|---|---|---|
| Anaphylactic | Infusion of IgA proteins to IgA-deficient recipient who has developed IgA antibody. | Anxiety, urticaria, wheezing, progressing to cyanosis, shock, possible cardiac arrest. | Do not restart transfusion if fever or pulmonary symptoms develop.<br>Initiate CPR, if indicated.<br>Have epinephrine ready for injection (0.4 ml of a 1:1000 solution subcutaneously or 0.1 ml of 1:1000 solution diluted to 10 ml with saline for IV use).<br>**Do not restart transfusion.** | Transfuse extensively washed RBC products, from which all plasma has been removed. Alternatively, use blood from IgA-deficient donor. |

| Circulatory overload | Fluid administered faster than the circulation can accommodate. | Cough, dyspnea, pulmonary congestion (rales), headache, hypertension, tachycardia, distended neck veins. | Place patient upright with feet in dependent position. Administer prescribed diuretics, oxygen, morphine. Phlebotomy may be indicated. | Adjust transfusion volume and flow rate based on patient size and clinical status. Have transfusion service divide unit into smaller aliquots for better spacing of fluid input. |
| Sepsis | Transfusion of contaminated blood components. | Rapid onset of chills, high fever, vomiting, diarrhea, and marked hypotension and shock. | Obtain culture of patient's blood and send bag with remaining blood to transfusion service for further study. Treat septicemia as directed—antibiotics, IV fluids, vasopressors, steroids. | Collect, process, store, and transfuse blood products according to blood banking standards and infuse within 4 hr of starting time. |

*IgA*, Immunoglobulin A; *CPR*, cardiopulmonary resuscitation.

expand all fluid compartments. Table 6-3 compares commonly prescribed crystalloid solutions.

*Colloids* are solutions that contain cells, proteins, or synthetic macromolecules that do not readily cross the capillary membrane. These solutions remain within the vascular space and, depending on their concentration, may cause an osmotic shift of fluids from the interstitum into the intravascular space. Table 6-4 compares commonly prescribed colloid solutions. Blood is the most commonly administered colloid. See Table 6-7 for common causes of blood transfusion reactions and the box on p. 81 for nursing management of transfusion reactions.

# Disorders of Sodium Balance

7

Sodium plays a vital role in maintaining concentration and volume of extracellular fluid (ECF). It is the main cation of ECF and the major determinant of ECF osmolality. Under normal conditions, ECF osmolality can be estimated by doubling the serum sodium value. Sodium imbalances usually are associated with parallel changes in osmolality. Sodium also is important in maintaining irritability and conduction of nerve and muscle tissue and assists with the regulation of acid-base balance.

## Sodium Changes

The average daily intake of sodium far exceeds the body's normal daily requirements. The kidneys are responsible for excreting the excess and are capable of conserving sodium avidly during periods of extreme sodium restriction. Three hormones are the primary regulators of renal sodium excretion. Both angiotensin II and aldosterone enhance renal sodium conservation. The major stimulus to the release of angiotensin II is a low ECF volume, and, in turn, aldosterone is released in response to increased angiotensin II. In contrast, atrial natriuretic factor increases renal excretion of sodium in response to ECF volume expansion.

Sodium concentration is maintained via regulation of water intake and excretion. If serum sodium is elevated (hypernatremia), serum osmolality increases, stimulating the thirst center and causing an increased release of antidiuretic hormone (ADH) by the posterior pituitary gland. ADH acts on the kidneys to conserve water. The combination of an increased water intake and renal water conservation help restore the normal sodium level. Conversely, when the serum sodium concentration is decreased (hyponatremia), the kidneys respond by excreting excess water. Changes in serum sodium levels typically reflect changes in water balance. Gains or losses of total body sodium are not necessarily reflected by the serum sodium level. Normal serum sodium levels are 135 to 145 mEq/L.

# Hyponatremia

Hyponatremia (serum sodium <135 mEq/L) can occur because of a net gain of water or loss of sodium-rich fluids that are replaced by water. Clinical indicators and treatment depend on the cause of hyponatremia and whether it is associated with a normal, decreased, or increased ECF volume. For more information, see pp. 215-216, pp. 218-219, and Chapters 22 and 25.

 ## Assessment

1. **Clinical manifestations:**
   Note: Neurologic symptoms usually do not occur until the serum sodium level has dropped to approximately 120 to 125 mEq/L.
   - *Hyponatremia with decreased ECF volume:* Irritability, apprehension, dizziness, personality changes, postural hypotension, dry mucous membranes, cold and clammy skin, tremors, seizures, and coma.
   - *Hyponatremia with normal or increased ECF volume:* Headache, lassitude, apathy, confusion, weakness, edema, weight gain, elevated blood pressure (BP), muscle cramps, convulsions, and coma.
2. **Hemodynamic measurements:**
   - *Decreased ECF volume:* Evidence of hypovolemia, including decreased central venous pressure (CVP), pulmonary artery pressure (PAP), cardiac output (CO), mean arterial pressure (MAP), and increased systemic vascular resistance (SVR).
   - *Increased ECF volume:* Evidence of hypervolemia, including increased CVP, PAP, and MAP.
3. **History and risk factors:**
   - *Decreased ECF volume:*
     —Gastrointestinal (GI) losses: Diarrhea, vomiting, fistulas, and nasogastric (NG) suction.
     —Renal losses: Diuretics, salt-wasting kidney disease, and adrenal insufficiency.
     —Skin losses: Burns and wound drainage.

■ *Normal/increased ECF volume:*
—Syndrome of inappropriate secretion of antidiuretic hormone (SIADH): Excessive production of ADH (see Chapter 20).
—Edematous states: Congestive heart failure, cirrhosis, and nephrotic syndrome.
—Excessive administration of hypotonic intravenous (IV) fluids.
—Oliguric renal failure.
—Primary psychogenic polydipsia.

NOTE: Hyperlipidemia, hyperproteinemia, and hyperglycemia may cause a pseudohyponatremia. Hyperlipidemia and hyperproteinemia reduce the total percentage of plasma that is water. The sodium/water ratio of the plasma does not change, but the plasma sodium level is reduced because there is a reduction in plasma water. With hyperglycemia, the osmotic action of the elevated glucose causes a shift of water out of the cells and into the ECF, thus diluting the existing sodium. For every 100 mg/dl glucose is elevated, sodium is diluted by 1.6 mEq/L.

## Diagnostic Tests

1. **Serum sodium:** Will be less than 135 mEq/L.
2. **Serum osmolality:** Decreased, except in cases of pseudohyponatremia, azotemia, or ingestion of toxins that increase osmolality (e.g., ethanol, methanol).
3. **Urine specific gravity:** Decreased because of the kidneys' attempt to excrete excess water. In patients with the SIADH, the urine is inappropriately concentrated.
4. **Urine sodium:** Decreased (usually <20 mEq/L) except in SIADH and adrenal insufficiency.

## Collaborative Management

The goal of therapy is to get the patient out of immediate danger (i.e., return sodium to >120 mEq/L) and then gradually return sodium to a normal level and restore normal ECF volume.

## Hyponatremia with Reduced Extracellular Fluid Volume

1. **Replacement of sodium and fluid losses.**
2. **Replacement of other electrolyte losses** (e.g., potassium, bicarbonate).

3. **IV hypertonic saline:** If serum sodium is dangerously low or the patient is very symptomatic. Used only until the patient's neurologic condition improves or a safe sodium level has been attained.

## Hyponatremia with Expanded Extracellular Fluid Volume

1. **Removal or treatment of the underlying cause**
2. **Loop diuretic** (thiazide diuretics should be avoided)
3. **Water restriction**
4. **Hemofiltration**

NOTE: Too-rapid correction of chronic hyponatremia may result in irreversible neurologic damage and death.

 ## Nursing Diagnoses and Interventions

**Fluid volume deficit** related to abnormal fluid loss; **fluid volume excess** related to excessive intake of hypotonic solutions or increased retention of water.

Desired outcomes: The patient is normovolemic as evidenced by heart rate (HR) 60 to 100 beats per minute (bpm), respiratory rate (RR) 12 to 20 breaths/min, BP within the patient's normal range, and CVP 2 to 6 mm Hg. For critical care patients, PAP is 20-30/8-15 mm Hg.

1. If the patient is receiving hypertonic saline, assess carefully for signs of intravascular fluid overload: tachypnea, tachycardia, shortness of breath (SOB), crackles, rhonchi, increased CVP, increased PAP, gallop rhythm, and increased BP. If given too rapidly, hypertonic saline may cause crenation (shriveling) of the red blood cells in addition to causing an osmotic shift of fluid into the vascular space.
2. For other interventions, see p. 65 for "fluid volume deficit"; see p. 70 for "fluid volume excess."

**Altered protection** related to neurosensory alterations secondary to a serum sodium level less than 120 to 125 mEq/L or too-rapid correction of hyponatremia.

Desired outcome: The patient verbalizes orientation to person, place, and time.

1. Assess and document level of consciousness (LOC), orientation, and neurologic status with each vital sign (VS) check. Reorient the patient as necessary. Alert the physician to significant changes.
2. Inform the patient and significant others that altered sensorium is temporary and will improve with treatment.

3. Keep side rails up and bed in lowest position, with wheels locked.
4. Use reality therapy such as clocks, calendars, and familiar objects; keep these items at the bedside within the patient's visual field.
5. If seizures are expected, pad side rails and keep appropriate-size airway at the bedside.
6. Monitor serum sodium levels. On the average, sodium levels should not increase at a rate greater than 0.5 to 1 mEq/L/hr in patients being treated for symptomatic hyponatremia because of the risk of neurologic damage. As well, levels should not increase at an *average* rate of more than 0.5 mEq/L/hr in patients without symptoms. The overall increase during the first 24 to 48 hours of treatment is more important than the individual hourly rate of increase.

## Patient-Family Teaching Guidelines

Give the patient and significant others verbal and written instructions for the following:

1. Medications, including drug name, purpose, dosage, frequency, precautions, and potential side effects. Teach signs and symptoms of hypokalemia if the patient is taking diuretics and provide examples of foods that are high in potassium (see the box on p. 100).
2. Fluid restriction, if prescribed. Teach the patient that a portion of fluid allotment can be taken as ice or Popsicles to minimize thirst.
3. Signs and symptoms of hypovolemia if hypernatremia is related to abnormal fluid losses.

## Hypernatremia

Hypernatremia (serum sodium level >145 mEq/L) may occur with water loss, water deprivation, or sodium gain. Because sodium is the major determinant of ECF osmolality, hypernatremia always causes hypertonicity. In turn, hypertonicity causes a shift of water out of the cells, which leads to cellular dehydration.

## Assessment

1. **Signs and symptoms:** Intense thirst, fatigue, restlessness, agitation, and coma. Symptomatic hypernatremia occurs only in individuals who do not have access to water or who

have an altered thirst mechanism (e.g., infants, the elderly, those who are comatose).

2. **Physical assessment:** Low-grade fever, flushed skin, peripheral and pulmonary edema (sodium gain); postural hypotension (water loss); and increased muscle tone and deep tendon reflexes.

3. **Hemodynamic measurements:** Variable.
   - *Sodium excess:* Increased CVP and PAP.
   - *Water loss:* Decreased CVP and PAP. The volume effects of water loss are minimized because of movement of water out of the cells secondary to hypernatremia-induced hypertonicity.

4. **History and risk factors:**
   - *Sodium gain:* IV administration of hypertonic saline or sodium bicarbonate, increased oral intake, primary aldosteronism, saltwater near-drowning, drugs such as sodium polystyrene sulfonate (Kayexalate).
   - *Water loss:* Increased insensible and sensible fluid loss (e.g., diaphoresis, respiratory infection), diabetes insipidus (see Chapter 20), or osmotic diuresis (e.g., hyperglycemia).

NOTE: Symptoms are most likely to develop with a sudden increase in plasma sodium. After approximately 24 hours, brain cells adjust to ECF hypertonicity by increasing intracellular osmolality. The exact mechanism by which this occurs is unclear, but it is known that this increased osmolality helps maintain cellular hydration. Thus individuals with chronic hypernatremia may exhibit few symptoms. This adaptive mechanism has great significance in the treatment of hypernatremia. If the plasma sodium is reduced too quickly via administration of water, there will be a rapid movement of water into the cells as a result of increased intracellular osmolality. The net result may be dangerous cerebral edema (see p. 22).

## Diagnostic Tests

1. **Serum sodium:** Will be greater than 145 mEq/L.
2. **Serum osmolality:** Increased because of elevated serum sodium.
3. **Urine specific gravity and osmolality:** Increased because of the kidneys' attempt to retain water; decreased in diabetes insipidus.

4. **Dehydration test:** Water is withheld for 16 to 18 hours. Serum and urine osmolality are then checked 1 hour after administration of ADH. This test is used to identify the etiology of polyuric syndromes (e.g., central versus nephrogenic diabetes insipidus).

## Collaborative Management

1. **IV or oral water replacement:** To treat water loss. If sodium is more than 160 mEq/L, IV $D_5W$ or hypotonic saline is given to replace pure water deficit.
2. **Diuretics in combination with oral or IV water replacement:** To treat sodium gain.

NOTE: Hypernatremia is corrected slowly, over approximately 2 days.

3. **Desmopressin acetate (DDAVP):** To treat central diabetes insipidus.
4. **Removal of cause** (e.g., medications such as lithium) in nephrogenic diabetes insipidus.

## Nursing Diagnoses and Interventions

*ndx:*

**Altered protection** related to altered sensorium secondary to primary hypernatremia or cerebral edema occurring with too-rapid correction of hypernatremia.

**Desired outcomes:** The patient verbalizes orientation to time, place, and person and does not exhibit evidence of injury as a result of altered sensorium or seizures.

1. Cerebral edema may occur if hypernatremia is corrected too rapidly. Monitor serial serum sodium levels; notify the physician of rapid decreases.
2. Assess the patient for indicators of cerebral edema: lethargy, headache, nausea, vomiting, increased BP, widening pulse pressure, decreased pulse rate, and seizures.
3. Assess and document LOC, orientation, and neurologic status with each check of VS. Reorient the patient as necessary. Alert the physician to significant changes.
4. Inform the patient and significant others that altered sensorium is temporary and will improve with treatment.
5. Keep side rails up and bed in lowest position, with wheels locked.
6. Use reality therapy such as clocks, calendars, and familiar

objects; keep these items at the bedside within the patient's visual field.

7. If seizures are anticipated, pad side rails and keep appropriate-size airway at the bedside.

8. Provide comfort measures to decrease thirst.

See p. 65 for fluid volume deficit (applicable to hypernatremia caused by water loss); see p. 70 for fluid volume excess (applicable to hypernatremia caused by sodium gain).

## Patient-Family Teaching Guidelines

Give the patient and significant others verbal and written instructions for the following:

1. Medications, including drug name, purpose, dosage, frequency, precautions, and potential side effects. Teach signs and symptoms of hypokalemia if the patient is taking diuretics and review foods that are high in potassium (see the box on p. 100).

2. Signs and symptoms of hypovolemia, if hypernatremia is related to abnormal fluid loss.

3. The importance of ensuring that infants and the elderly are given adequate water to replace normal and abnormal losses (e.g., during hot weather).

# Disorders of Potassium Balance

**8**

Potassium is the primary intracellular cation, and it plays a vital role in cell metabolism. A relatively small amount (approximately 2%) of potassium is located within the extracellular fluid (ECF) and is maintained within a narrow range. The vast majority of the body's potassium is located within the cells. The sodium-potassium adenosine triphosphatase (ATPase) pump located in the cell membrane is critical to maintaining the balance between intracellular and extracellular potassium. The pump actively transports sodium out of the cell and potassium into the cell. Adequate intracellular magnesium is required for normal function of the pump. Because the ratio of intracellular fluid (ICF) to ECF potassium helps determine the resting membrane potential of nerve and muscle cells, an alteration in the plasma potassium level may adversely affect neuromuscular and cardiac function.

Distribution of potassium between ECF and ICF is affected by ECF pH, as well as by several hormones, including insulin, epinephrine, and aldosterone. Increases in these hormones cause an increased movement of potassium into the cells. Acute changes in serum pH are accompanied by reciprocal changes in serum potassium concentration. In acidosis, for example, excess hydrogen ions move into the cells to be buffered. To maintain electric neutrality within the cell, another positive ion (e.g., potassium) must move out. In alkalosis the reverse occurs. Hydrogen ions shift out of the cell and potassium ions shift in to replace them.

The body gains potassium through foods (primarily meats, fruits, and vegetables) and medications. In addition, ECF gains potassium any time there is a breakdown of cells (tissue catabolism) or movement of potassium out of the cells. However, an elevated serum potassium level usually does not occur unless there is a concomitant reduction in renal function. Potassium is lost from the body through the kidneys, gastrointestinal (GI) tract, and skin. Potassium may be lost from ECF because of an intracellular shift or tissue anabolism.

The kidneys are the primary regulators of potassium balance. They do this by adjusting the amount of potassium that is excreted in the urine. As the serum potassium level rises after a potassium load, so does the level in the renal tubular cell. This creates a concentration gradient favoring the movement of potassium into the renal tubule with the loss of potassium in the urine. The presence of aldosterone also increases the excretion of potassium. Thus conditions that increase aldosterone levels (e.g., administration of corticosteroids or postsurgical stress) may increase urinary excretion of potassium. The rate of urine flow also affects potassium excretion, so that conditions associated with increased urine production may increase potassium loss. The kidneys are unable to conserve potassium as avidly as sodium, and a significant amount of potassium still may be lost in the urine in the presence of potassium depletion. Normal serum potassium is 3.5 to 5 mEq/L.

# Hypokalemia

Hypokalemia occurs because of a loss of potassium from the body or a movement of potassium into the cells and is rarely the result of inadequate intake alone. Hypomagnesemia may contribute to the development of hypokalemia as a result of increased movement of potassium out of cells and increased urinary excretion. NOTE: Changes in serum potassium levels reflect changes in ECF potassium, not necessarily changes in total body levels.

## Assessment

1. **Clinical manifestations:** Fatigue, muscle weakness, leg cramps, soft and flabby muscles, nausea, vomiting, ileus, paresthesias, enhanced digitalis effect, and decreased urine concentration (e.g., with polyuria).
2. **Physical assessment:** Decreased bowel sounds caused by smooth muscle weakness, weak and irregular pulse, decreased reflexes, and decreased muscle tone.
3. **History and risk factors:**
   - *Reduction in total body potassium:*
     —Hyperaldosteronism (e.g., congenital adrenal hyperplasia).

—Diuretics or abnormal urinary losses.

—Increased GI losses, especially gastric losses (e.g., pyloric stenosis).

—Increased loss through diaphoresis.

NOTE: Poor dietary intake may contribute to, but rarely will cause, hypokalemia. Hypokalemia may develop in the patient who is maintained on parenteral fluids with inadequate replacement of potassium.

- ■ *Intracellular shift:*

—Increased insulin (e.g., from total parenteral nutrition [TPN]).

—Alkalosis or after correction of acidosis (e.g., treatment of diabetic ketoacidosis [DKA]).

—During periods of tissue repair after burns, trauma, or starvation. Usually, this is accompanied by inadequate intake or replacement of potassium.

—Administration of beta-adrenergic agonists (e.g., terbutaline, dobutamine) or increased beta-adrenergic activity (e.g., stress, coronary ischemia).

## Diagnostic Tests

1. **Serum potassium:** Values will be less than 3.5 mEq/L.
2. **Arterial blood gases (ABGs):** May show metabolic alkalosis (increased pH and bicarbonate ion [$HCO_3^-$]) because hypokalemia usually is associated with this condition.
3. **Electrocardiogram (ECG):** ST-segment depression, flattened T wave, presence of U wave, and ventricular dysrhythmias (Figure 8-1). NOTE: Hypokalemia potentiates the effects of digitalis. ECG may reveal signs of digitalis toxicity in spite of a normal serum digitalis level.

## Collaborative Management

1. **Treatment of the underlying cause.**
2. **Replacement of potassium:** Either by mouth (PO) (via increased dietary intake or medication) or intravenously (IV). The usual dose is 40 to 80 mEq/day in divided doses. IV potassium is necessary if hypokalemia is severe or the patient is unable to take potassium orally. IV potassium should not be administered at rates exceeding 10 to 20 mEq/hr or in concentrations higher than 30 to 40 mEq/L unless hypokalemia is severe because this can result in life-threatening hyperkalemia. If potassium is administered

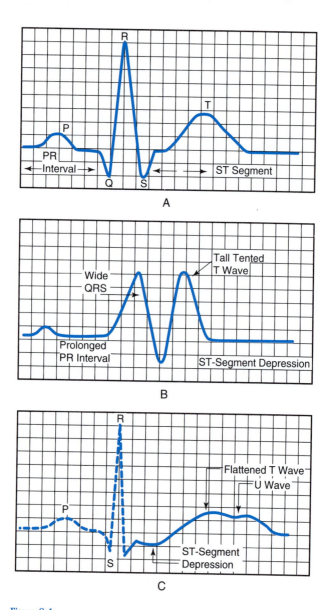

Figure 8-1
A, Normal electrocardiographic tracing. B, Serum potassium level above normal. C, Serum potassium level below normal.

via a peripheral line, the rate of administration may need to be reduced to prevent irritation of vessels. Patients receiving 10 to 20 mEq/hr should be on a continuous cardiac monitor. The development of peaked T waves suggests the presence of hyperkalemia and requires immediate physician notification. Potassium never may be given as an IV push.

Potassium is usually replaced in combination with chloride or phosphate. Because hypokalemia is frequently associated with ECF volume deficit and chloride loss (e.g., vomiting or diuretics), potassium chloride is usually the preparation of choice. When hypokalemia is associated with a need for intracellular anions (e.g., TPN or treatment of DKA), potassium phosphate may be the preferred preparation. In the treatment of DKA, when large volumes of isotonic sodium chloride are given, the phosphate preparation has the additional benefit of avoiding additional chloride administration.

3. **Potassium-sparing diuretics:** May be given in place of oral potassium supplements.

4. **Potassium chloride salt substitute:** May be used to supplement potassium intake (1 teaspoon equals approximately 60 mEq potassium chloride).

## Nursing Diagnoses and Interventions

**Decreased cardiac output** related to altered conduction (risk of ventricular dysrhythmias) secondary to hypokalemia or too-rapid correction of hypokalemia with resulting hyperkalemia.

**Desired outcomes:** ECG shows normal configuration and absence of ventricular dysrhythmias. Pulse rate and rhythm are normal for the patient. Serum potassium levels are within the normal range (3.5 to 5 mEq/L).

1. Administer IV potassium supplement as prescribed. Avoid giving IV potassium chloride at a rate faster than recommended because this can lead to life-threatening hyperkalemia (see p. 97). Potassium supplementation for symptomatic hypokalemia is usually given in isotonic saline because $D_5W$ will increase insulin-induced intracellular shift of potassium. Do not add potassium chloride to IV solution containers in the hanging position because this can cause layering of the medication. Instead, invert the solution container before adding the medication and mix well. NOTE: IV potassium

chloride can cause local irritation of veins and chemical phlebitis. Assess IV insertion site for erythema, heat, or pain. Consult with the physician if symptoms develop. Irritation may be relieved by applying an ice bag, giving mild sedation, or numbing insertion site with a small amount of local anesthetic. Phlebitis may necessitate changing the IV site.

2. Administer oral potassium supplements as prescribed. NOTE: Oral supplements may cause GI irritation. Administer with a full glass of water or fruit juice; encourage the patient to sip slowly. Consult with the physician if symptoms of abdominal pain, distention, nausea, or vomiting develop. Do not switch potassium supplements without physician's prescription.

3. Encourage intake of foods high in potassium (see the box below). Salt substitutes may be used as an inexpensive potassium supplement.

4. Monitor intake and output (I&O) hourly. Alert the physician to urine output of less than 0.5 ml/kg/hr. Unless severe, symptomatic hypokalemia is present, potassium supplements should not be given if the patient has an inadequate urine output because hyperkalemia can develop rapidly in patients with oliguria (<15 to 20 ml/hr). Alert the physician to elevated blood urea nitrogen (BUN) or creatinine levels.

5. Monitor for the presence of an irregular pulse or pulse deficit (a discrepancy between the apical and radial pulse rates). Alert the physician to changes.

## Foods High in Potassium

| | |
|---|---|
| Apricots | Nuts |
| Artichokes | Oranges, orange juice |
| Avocado | Potatoes |
| Banana | Prune juice |
| Cantaloupe | Pumpkin |
| Carrots | Rhubarb |
| Chocolate | Salt substitute |
| Dried beans, peas | Spinach |
| Dried fruit | Swiss chard |
| Meat | Sweet potatoes |
| Melons | Tomatoes, tomato juice, tomato sauce |
| Mushrooms | Turnips |

6. Physical indicators of abnormal potassium levels are difficult to identify in the patient who is critically ill. Monitor ECG for signs of continuing hypokalemia (ST-segment depression, flattened T wave, presence of U wave, ventricular dysrhythmias) or hyperkalemia (tall, thin T waves; prolonged PR interval; ST depression; widened QRS; loss of P wave), which may develop during potassium replacement (see Figure 8-1).

7. Monitor serum potassium levels carefully, especially in individuals at risk for developing hypokalemia such as patients taking diuretics or receiving nasogastric suction.

8. Administer potassium cautiously in patients receiving potassium-sparing diuretics (e.g., spironolactone amiloride, or triamterene) or ACE inhibitors (e.g., captopril) because of the potential for the development of hyperkalemia.

9. Because hypokalemia can potentiate the effects of digitalis, monitor patients receiving digitalis for signs of increased digitalis effect: multifocal or bigeminal premature ventricular contractions (PVCs), paroxysmal atrial tachycardia with varying atrioventricular (AV) block, and other heart blocks.

**Ineffective breathing pattern** (or risk for same) related to weakness or paralysis of respiratory muscles secondary to *severe* hypokalemia (potassium <2 to 2.5 mEq/L).

**Desired outcome:** The patient has effective breathing pattern as evidenced by normal respiratory depth, pattern, and rate of 12 to 20 breaths/min.

1. If the patient is exhibiting signs of worsening hypokalemia, be aware that severe hypokalemia can lead to weakness of respiratory muscles, resulting in shallow respirations and eventually, apnea and respiratory arrest. Assess character, rate, and depth of respirations. Alert the physician promptly if respirations become rapid and shallow.

2. Keep manual resuscitator at the patient's bedside if severe hypokalemia is suspected.

3. Reposition the patient every 2 hours to prevent stasis of secretions; suction airway as needed.

## Patient-Family Teaching Guidelines

Give the patient and significant others verbal and written instructions for the following:

1. Medications, including name, purpose, dosage, frequency,

precautions, and potential side effects. Teach the patient the importance of taking prescribed potassium supplements if taking diuretics or digitalis. Review the indicators of digitalis toxicity.

2. Indicators of hypokalemia and hyperkalemia.

3. Foods that are high in potassium (see the box on p. 100); use of salt substitute to supplement potassium, if appropriate.

# Hyperkalemia

Hyperkalemia (serum potassium level >5 mEq/L) occurs because of an increased intake of potassium, a decreased urinary excretion of potassium, or movement of potassium out of the cells. Note: Changes in serum potassium levels reflect changes in ECF potassium not necessarily changes in total body levels. In diabetic ketoacidosis, for example, a large quantity of potassium may be lost in the urine as a result of the glucose-induced osmotic diuresis. Although there may be a significant reduction in total body potassium levels, the patient initially may present with a normal or elevated potassium. This occurs because of the shift of potassium out of the cells secondary to lack of insulin, increased tissue catabolism, and acidosis. For additional information, see Chapter 20. Chronic hyperkalemia is usually the result of decreased urinary excretion of potassium.

## Assessment

1. **Clinical manifestations:** Irritability, anxiety, abdominal cramping, diarrhea, weakness (especially of lower extremities), and paresthesias.

2. **Physical assessment:** Irregular pulse; cardiac standstill if hyperkalemia is sudden or severe.

3. **History and risk factors:**
   - *Inappropriately high intake of potassium:* Usually, IV potassium delivery.
   - *Decreased excretion of potassium:* For example, with renal disease, use of potassium-sparing diuretics or ACE inhibitors, or adrenal insufficiency (Addison's disease).
   - *Movement of potassium out of the cells:* For example, with acidosis, insulin deficiency, and tissue catabolism (e.g., occurring with fever, sepsis, trauma, or surgery).

NOTE: The severity of symptoms depends on the rate of change in the serum potassium level as well as the overall level.

## Diagnostic Tests

1. **Serum potassium:** Will be more than 5 mEq/L. NOTE: Several factors may cause a falsely high serum potassium because of increased release of intracellular potassium in the laboratory specimen (e.g., a high platelet count, prolonged use of a tourniquet at the time of venipuncture, hemolysis of the blood specimen, or delayed separation of plasma and cells).
2. **ABGs:** May show metabolic acidosis (decreased pH and $HCO_3^-$) because hyperkalemia often occurs with acidosis.
3. **Diagnostic ECG:** Progressive changes include tall, thin T waves; prolonged PR interval; ST depression; widened QRS; loss of P wave. Eventually, QRS becomes widened further and cardiac arrest occurs (see Figure 8-1).
4. **Urine potassium:** May be helpful in the diagnosis of Addison's disease.

## Collaborative Management

The goal is to treat the underlying cause and return the serum potassium level to normal.

## Subacute

1. **Cation exchange resins (e.g., Kayexalate):** Given either orally, nasogastrically, or via retention enema to exchange sodium for potassium in the bowel. The solution is usually combined with sorbitol to prevent constipation from the Kayexalate and induce diarrhea, thus increasing potassium loss in the bowels. Resins have a faster onset of action when given rectally. NOTE: Kayexalate may bind with other cations in the GI tract and contribute to the development of hypomagnesemia or hypocalcemia.
2. **Reduced potassium intake:** A diet avoiding high potassium content foods (see the box on p. 100). Special IV or enteral formulas are available for patients with renal failure.

## Acute

1. **IV calcium gluconate:** To counteract the neuromuscular and cardiac effects of hyperkalemia. Serum potassium levels will

remain elevated. Calcium chloride may also be used. NOTE: Calcium chloride and calcium gluconate are *not* interchangeable. Although both come in 10-ml ampules, calcium gluconate contains only 4.5 mEq of calcium, whereas calcium chloride contains 13.6 mEq of calcium.

2. **IV glucose and insulin:** To shift potassium into the cells. This reduces serum potassium temporarily (approximately 6 hours). Usually hypertonic glucose (either an amp of $D_{50}W$ or 250 to 500 ml of $D_{10}W$) is given with regular insulin.

3. **Sodium bicarbonate:** To shift potassium into the cells. Reduces serum potassium temporarily (for approximately 1 to 2 hours). NOTE: The effects of calcium, glucose and insulin, and sodium bicarbonate are temporary. Usually it is necessary to follow these medications with a therapy that removes potassium from the body, for example, dialysis or administration of cation exchange resins.

4. **Dialysis:** To remove potassium from the body. Dialysis is the most effective means of removing excess potassium.

## Nursing Diagnoses and Interventions

**Decreased cardiac output** (or risk for same) related to altered conduction (risk of ventricular dysrhythmias) secondary to severe hyperkalemia or too-rapid correction of hyperkalemia with resulting hypokalemia.

**Desired outcomes:** ECG shows no evidence of ventricular dysrhythmias related to hypokalemia (U wave, PVCs) or hyperkalemia (peaked T wave). Serum potassium levels are within the normal range (3.5 to 5 mEq/L).

1. Monitor I&O. Consult with the physician for urine output less than 0.5 ml/kg/hr. Oliguria increases the risk for developing hyperkalemia.

2. Monitor for indicators for hyperkalemia (e.g., irritability, anxiety, abdominal cramping, diarrhea, weakness of lower extremities, paresthesias, irregular pulse). Also be alert to indicators of hypokalemia (e.g., fatigue, muscle weakness, leg cramps, nausea, vomiting, decreased bowel sounds, paresthesias, weak and irregular pulse) following treatment. Assess for hidden sources of potassium: medications (e.g., potassium penicillin G), banked blood (the older the blood, the greater the amount of potassium because of the release

of potassium as red blood cells that die and break down), salt substitute, GI bleeding, or conditions causing increased catabolism such as infection or trauma.

3. Monitor serum potassium levels, especially in patients at risk of developing hyperkalemia such as individuals with renal failure. Notify the physician of levels above or below the normal range.

4. Physical indicators of abnormal potassium levels are difficult to identify in the patient who is critically ill. Monitor ECG for signs of hypokalemia (ST-segment depression, flattened T waves, presence of U wave, ventricular dysrhythmias), which may develop secondary to therapy, or continuing hyperkalemia (tall, thin T waves; prolonged PR interval; ST depression; widened QRS; loss of P wave). Notify the physician *stat* if ECG changes occur. ECG changes at a given potassium level will be less dramatic in the chronic renal patient who develops hyperkalemia more slowly. See Figure 8-1 for ECG changes with hypokalemia and hyperkalemia.

5. Administer calcium gluconate as prescribed, giving it cautiously in patients receiving digitalis because digitalis toxicity can occur. NOTE: Do not add calcium gluconate to solutions containing sodium bicarbonate because precipitates may form. However, IV glucose and sodium bicarbonate ($NaHCO_3$) may be combined without harmful precipitate. Insulin should be given separately. For more information about calcium administration, see p. 111.

6. If administering cation exchange resins by enema, encourage the patient to retain the solution for at least 30 to 60 minutes to ensure therapeutic effects. Administer kayexalate (without sorbitol) via a Foley catheter inserted into the rectum. The balloon is filled with sterile water to keep the catheter in place, and the catheter is clamped. Cleansing enemas are recommended before administration to enhance absorption and afterward to reduce the risk of bowel complications. Follow specific institution policy.

7. Administer insulin and glucose in the order prescribed. When glucose is administered first, it stimulates endogenous insulin release and may potentiate the potassium-lowering effect of the exogenous insulin.

Patient-Family Teaching Guidelines

Give the patient and significant others verbal and written instructions for the following:

1. Medications, including name, purpose, dosage, frequency, precautions, and potential side effects.

2. Indicators of both hypokalemia and hyperkalemia. Alert the patient to the following signs and symptoms that necessitate immediate medical attention: weakness or pulse irregularities. Teach the patient and significant others how to measure pulse rate and detect irregularities.

3. Foods high in potassium, which should be avoided (see the box on p. 100). Remind the patient that salt substitute and "Lite" salt also should be avoided. Fruits that are relatively low in potassium include apples, grapes, and cranberries.

4. Importance of preventing recurrent hyperkalemia; review potential causes.

# Disorders of Calcium Balance

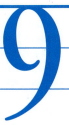

Calcium, one of the body's most abundant ions, primarily is combined with phosphorus to form the mineral salts of the bones and teeth. In addition, calcium exerts a sedative effect on nerve cells and has important intracellular functions, including development of the cardiac action potential and contraction of muscles. Less than 1% of the body's calcium is contained within extracellular fluid (ECF), yet this concentration is regulated carefully by parathyroid hormone, metabolites of vitamin D, and calcitonin. Parathyroid hormone is released by the parathyroid gland in response to a low serum calcium level. It increases resorption of bone (movement of calcium and phosphorus out of the bone); activates vitamin D, which increases the absorption of calcium from the gastrointestinal (GI) tract; and stimulates the kidneys to conserve calcium and excrete phosphorus. Calcitonin is produced by the thyroid gland when serum calcium levels are elevated. It inhibits bone resorption.

The ECF gains calcium from intestinal absorption of dietary calcium and resorption of bones. It is lost from the ECF via secretion into the GI tract, urinary excretion, and deposition in the bone; a small amount is lost in sweat.

Calcium is present in three different forms in the plasma: ionized, bound, and complexed. Approximately half of the plasma calcium is free, ionized calcium. Slightly less than half the plasma calcium is bound to protein, primarily to albumin. The remaining small percentage is combined with nonprotein anions such as phosphate, citrate, and carbonate. Only the ionized calcium is physiologically important. The percentage of calcium that is ionized is affected by plasma pH, phosphorus, and albumin levels. Therefore these factors must be considered when evaluating total calcium levels.

The relationship between ionized calcium and plasma pH is reciprocal: an increase in pH decreases the percentage of calcium that is ionized. Patients with alkalosis (an increased pH), for example, may show signs of hypocalcemia despite a normal total calcium level (bound, complexed, and ionized). The relationship between plasma phosphorus and ionized calcium is also reciprocal. Changes in the plasma albumin level will affect the total serum calcium level without changing the level of free calcium. In hypoalbuminemia, less protein is available to bind with calcium and the total calcium level drops; however, the level of ionized calcium is unchanged.

## Hypocalcemia

Symptomatic hypocalcemia may occur because of a reduction of total body calcium or a reduction of the percentage of calcium that is ionized. Total calcium levels may be decreased as a result of increased calcium loss, reduced intake secondary to altered intestinal absorption, or altered regulation (e.g., hypoparathyroidism). Elevated phosphorus levels and decreased magnesium levels may precipitate hypocalcemia. Calcium and phosphorus have a reciprocal relationship: as one goes up, the other tends to go down. Hypomagnesemia may cause hypocalcemia as a result of the decreased action of the parathyroid hormone.

NOTE: The most common cause of a low total calcium level is hypoalbuminemia. However, if the level of ionized calcium remains normal, the condition is asymptomatic and no treatment is required. In the presence of a decreased serum albumin level, treatment should be based on ionized calcium levels.

### Assessment

1. **Clinical manifestations:** Numbness with tingling of fingers and circumoral region, hyperactive reflexes, muscle cramps, tetany, and convulsions. Lethargy and poor feeding may be present in the newborn. In chronic hypocalcemia, fractures may be present as a result of bone porosity.
2. **Physical assessment:**
   - *Positive Trousseau's sign:* Ischemia-induced carpal spasm. It is elicited by applying a blood pressure (BP) cuff to the upper arm and inflating it past systolic BP for 2 to 3 minutes.
   - *Positive Chvostek's sign:* Unilateral contraction of facial and eyelid muscles. It is elicited by irritating the facial nerve by percussing the face just in front of the ear.

3. **Electrocardiogram (ECG) changes:** Prolonged QT interval caused by elongation of ST segment; may develop a form of ventricular tachycardia: Torsades de pointes.
4. **History and risk factors:**
   - *Decreased ionized calcium:* For example, that occurring with alkalosis, administration of large quantities of citrated blood (citrate added to the blood to prevent clotting may bind with calcium, causing hypocalcemia), and hemodilution (e.g., caused by volume replacement with normal saline after hemorrhage).
   - *Increased calcium loss in body fluids:* For example, with certain diuretics.
   - *Decreased intestinal absorption:* For example, with decreased intake, impaired vitamin D metabolism (e.g., in renal failure), chronic diarrhea, and postgastrectomy.
   - *Hypoparathyroidism:* Congenital or acquired.
   - *Hyperphosphatemia:* For example, in renal failure.
   - *Hypomagnesemia.*
   - *Acute pancreatitis.*
   - *Chronic alcoholism.*

## Diagnostic Tests

1. **Total serum calcium level:** May be less than 8.5 mg/dl. Serum calcium levels should be evaluated with serum albumin. For every 1 g/dl drop in the serum albumin level, there is a 0.8 to 1 mg/dl drop in total calcium level.
2. **Ionized serum calcium:** Will be less than 4.5 mg/dl.
3. **Parathyroid hormone:** Decreased levels occur in hypoparathyroidism; increased levels may occur with other causes of hypocalcemia. Normal range is 150 to 350 pg/ml (varies among laboratories).
4. **Magnesium and phosphorus levels:** May be checked to identify potential causes of hypocalcemia.

## Collaborative Management

1. **Treatment of the underlying cause.**
2. **Calcium replacement:** Hypocalcemia is treated with oral (PO) or intravenous (IV) calcium. Tetany in the adult is treated with 10 to 20 ml of 10% calcium gluconate IV or a continuous drip of 100 ml of 10% calcium gluconate in 1000 ml $D_5W$, infused over at least 4 hours.

Table 9-1   Vitamin D prepartions

| Generic Name | Trade Name | Chemical Abbreviation |
|---|---|---|
| Calcifediol | Calderol | $25(OH)D_3$ |
| Calcitriol | Rocaltrol | $1,25(OH)_2D_3$ |
| | Calcijex | |
| Cholecalciferol | Delta D | $D_3$ |
| | Vitamin $D_3$ | |
| Dihydrotachysterol | Hytakerol | DHT |
| Ergocalciferol | Calciferol | $D_2$ |
| | Vitamin D | |
| | Deltalin Gelseals | |

3. **Magnesium replacement in individuals with magnesium deficiency.** Hypomagnesemia-induced hypocalcemia is often refractory to calcium therapy alone.
4. **Vitamin D therapy (e.g., dihydrotachysterol, calcitriol):** To increase calcium absorption from the GI tract (Table 9-1).
5. **Aluminum hydroxide antacids or calcium acetate:** To reduce an elevated phosphorus level before treating hypocalcemia.
6. **Increased dietary intake of calcium:** At least 1000 to 1500 mg/day in the adult.
7. **Oral calcium supplements such as calcium carbonate.**

_ndx_ ## Nursing Diagnoses and Interventions

**Altered protection** (risk of tetany and seizures) related to neurosensory alterations secondary to severe hypocalcemia.
**Desired outcomes:** The patient does not exhibit evidence of injury caused by complications of severe hypocalcemia. Serum calcium levels are within normal range (8.5 to 10.5 mg/dl).

1. Monitor the patient for evidence of worsening hypocalcemia: numbness and tingling of fingers and circumoral region, hyperactive reflexes, and muscle cramps. Consult with the physician promptly if these symptoms develop because they occur before overt tetany. In addition, consult with the physician if the patient has positive Trousseau's or Chvostek's signs because they also signal latent tetany. Monitor total and ionized calcium levels as available.

## Foods High in Calcium Content

| | |
|---|---|
| Cottage cheese | Seafood, especially canned |
| Cheese | sardines and canned salmon |
| Milk and cream | Rhubarb |
| Eggnog | Brazil nuts |
| Yogurt | Sesame seeds |
| Soy flour | Broccoli |
| Oat flakes | Collard, mustard, and turnip |
| Milk chocolate | greens |
| Ice cream | Spinach |
| Molasses | Tofu |

2. Administer IV calcium with caution. IV calcium should not be given faster than 0.5 to 1 ml/min because rapid administration can cause hypotension. Observe IV insertion site for evidence of infiltration because calcium will slough tissue. Concentrated calcium solutions should be administered through a central line. Do not add calcium to solutions containing bicarbonate or phosphate because precipitates will form. Digitalis toxicity may develop in patients taking digitalis because calcium potentiates its effects. Monitor the patient for signs and symptoms of hypercalcemia: lethargy, confusion, irritability, nausea, and vomiting. NOTE: Always clarify type of IV calcium to be given. Both calcium chloride and calcium gluconate come in 10-ml ampules. One ampule of calcium chloride contains approximately 13.6 mEq of calcium, whereas 1 ampule of calcium gluconate contains 4.5 mEq of calcium.

3. For patients with chronic hypocalcemia, administer PO calcium supplements and vitamin D preparations (see Table 9-1) as prescribed. Administer PO calcium 30 minutes before meals and/or at bedtime for maximal absorption. Administer aluminum hydroxide antacids or calcium acetate tablets (PhosLo) with meals to ensure phosphorus binding.

4. Encourage intake of foods high in calcium: milk products, meats, and leafy green vegetables (see the box above).

5. Notify the physician if response to calcium therapy is ineffective. Tetany that does not respond to IV calcium may be caused by hypomagnesemia.

6. Keep symptomatic patients on seizure precautions; decrease environmental stimuli.
7. Avoid hyperventilation in patients in whom hypocalcemia is suspected. Respiratory alkalosis may precipitate tetany as a result of increased pH with a reduction in ionized calcium.

**Decreased cardiac output** related to altered conduction or decreased cardiac contractility secondary to hypocalcemia or digitalis toxicity occurring with calcium replacement therapy.

Desired outcomes: The patient's cardiac output is adequate as evidenced by central venous pressure (CVP) 6 mm Hg or lower (≤12 cm $H_2O$), heart rate (HR) 100 beats per minute (bpm) or lower, BP within the patient's normal range, and absence of the clinical signs of heart failure or pulmonary edema (e.g., crackles, shortness of breath [SOB]). Critical care patients exhibit a pulmonary artery pressure (PAP) of 20-30/8-15 mm Hg.

1. Monitor ECG for signs of worsening hypocalcemia (prolonged QT interval) or digitalis toxicity with calcium replacement: multifocal or bigeminal premature ventricular contractions (PVC), paroxysmal atrial tachycardia with varying atrioventricular (AV) block, and other heart blocks.
2. Hypocalcemia may decrease cardiac contractility. Monitor the patient for signs of heart failure or pulmonary edema: crackles (rales), rhonchi, SOB, decreased BP, increased HR, increased PAP, or increased CVP.

**Ineffective breathing pattern** related to laryngeal spasm occurring with severe hypocalcemia.

Desired outcome: The patient exhibits respiratory depth, pattern, and rate (12 to 20 breaths/min) within normal range and is asymptomatic of laryngeal spasm: laryngeal stridor, dyspnea, or crowing.

1. Assess the patient's respiratory rate, character, and rhythm. Be alert to laryngeal stridor, dyspnea, and crowing, which occur with laryngeal spasm, a life-threatening complication of hypocalcemia.
2. Keep an emergency tracheostomy tray at the bedside of symptomatic patients.

## Patient-Family Teaching Guidelines

Give the patient and significant others verbal and written instructions for the following:

1. Medications, including drug name, purpose, dosage, frequency, precautions, and potential side effects.
2. Indicators of hypercalcemia and hypocalcemia. Review the symptoms that necessitate immediate medical attention: numbness and tingling of fingers and circumoral region and muscle cramps.
3. Foods that are high in calcium (see Table 9-1). NOTE: Many foods that are high in calcium, such as milk products, also are high in phosphorus and may need to be limited in patients with renal failure. A program of phosphorus control and calcium supplementation may be necessary for patients who have renal failure.

# Hypercalcemia

Symptomatic hypercalcemia can occur because of an increase in total serum calcium or an increase in the percentage of free, ionized calcium. If hypercalcemia is accompanied by a normal or elevated serum phosphorus level, calcium phosphate crystals may precipitate in the serum and deposit throughout the body. Soft tissue calcifications usually occur when the product (i.e., calcium × phosphorus) of the serum calcium and serum phosphorus exceeds 70 mg/dl. The most common causes of hypercalcemia are primary hyperparathyroidism and malignancy.

## Assessment

1. **Clinical manifestations:** Lethargy, weakness, anorexia, nausea, vomiting, polyuria, itching, bone pain, fractures, flank pain (secondary to renal calculi), depression, confusion, paresthesias, personality changes, stupor, and coma.
2. **ECG findings:** Shortening of ST segment and QT interval. PR interval is sometimes prolonged. Ventricular dysrhythmias can occur with severe hypercalcemia. There is an increased risk of digitalis toxicity.
3. **History and risk factors:**
   - *Increased intake of calcium:* Excessive administration during cardiopulmonary arrest.
   - *Increased intestinal absorption:* For example, with vitamin D or A overdose or hyperparathyroidism.
   - *Increased release of calcium from bone:* Occurs with

hyperparathyroidism, malignancies, prolonged immobilization, and Paget's disease.
- *Decreased urinary excretion:* Renal failure and certain medications (e.g., thiazide diuretics).
- *Increased ionized calcium:* Acidosis.

## Diagnostic Tests

1. **Total serum calcium level:** May be greater than 10.5 mg/dl. The total calcium level should be evaluated with the serum albumin level. For a 1 g/dl drop in serum albumin level, there will be a 0.8 to 1 mg/dl drop in total serum calcium.
2. **Ionized calcium:** Will be more than 5.5 mg/dl.
3. **Parathyroid hormone:** Increased levels occur in primary or secondary hyperparathyroidism.
4. **X-ray findings:** May reveal presence of osteoporosis, bone cavitation, or urinary calculi.

## Collaborative Management

NOTE: Mild, asymptomatic hypercalcemia often requires no treatment. Treatment of moderate hypercalcemia may depend on the severity of symptoms. Severe hypercalcemia (calcium levels >13.5 mg/dl) requires immediate treatment.

1. **Treatment of the underlying cause:** Antitumor chemotherapy for malignancy or partial parathyroidectomy for hyperparathyroidism; discontinuation of calcium supplements, vitamins A and D, and thiazide diuretics.
2. **IV normal saline:** Administered rapidly to increase urinary calcium excretion. Concomitant administration of furosemide prevents the development of fluid volume excess and further increases urinary calcium excretion.
3. **Low-calcium diet and cortisone:** To reduce intestinal absorption of calcium. Steroids compete with vitamin D, thereby reducing intestinal absorption of calcium. For a list of foods high in calcium, see the box on p. 111.
4. **Pamidronate or etidronate:** Bisphosphates that inhibit bone resorption.
5. **Plicamycin:** A cytotoxic antibiotic that acts directly on bone to reduce bone resorption. It is used primarily to treat hypercalcemia associated with neoplastic disease.
6. **Calcitonin:** To reduce bone resorption, increase bone deposition of calcium and phosphorus, and increase urinary

calcium and phosphate excretion. Skin testing for allergy may be necessary before administration of salmon calcitonin.

7. **Gallium nitrate:** Inhibits osteoclasts and increases bone calcium. It is used in the treatment of malignancy-induced hypercalcemia.

8. **Oral phosphates:** Used to treat mild hypercalcemia caused by primary hyperparathyroidism.

## Nursing Diagnoses and Interventions

**Altered protection** related to neuromuscular changes secondary to hypercalcemia.

**Desired outcomes:** The patient does not exhibit evidence of injury caused by neuromuscular or sensorium changes. The patient verbalizes orientation to person, place, and time. Serum calcium levels are within normal range (8.5 to 10.5 mg/dl).

1. Monitor the patient for worsening hypercalcemia. Assess and document the level of consciousness (LOC); the patient's orientation to person, place, and time; and neurologic status with each vital sign (VS) check.

2. Personality changes, hallucinations, paranoia, and memory loss may occur with hypercalcemia. Inform the patient and significant others that altered sensorium is temporary and will improve with treatment. Use reality therapy such as clocks, calendars, and familiar objects; keep them at the bedside within the patient's visual field.

3. Hypercalcemia causes neuromuscular depression with poor coordination, weakness, and altered gait. Provide a safe environment. Keep the side rails up and bed in the lowest position, with wheels locked. Assist the patient with ambulation if it is allowed.

4. Because hypercalcemia potentiates the effects of digitalis, monitor the patient taking digitalis for signs and symptoms of digitalis toxicity: anorexia, nausea, vomiting, and irregular pulse. ECG changes may include multifocal or bigeminal PVCs, paroxysmal atrial tachycardia with varying AV block, and other heart blocks. Monitor the patient for pulse changes in the non-ECG monitored setting.

5. Monitor the serum electrolyte values for changes in serum calcium (normal range is 8.5 to 10.5 mg/dl); potassium (normal range is 3.5 to 5 mEq/L); and phosphorus (normal

range is 2.5 to 4.5 mg/dl) secondary to therapy. Consult the physician for abnormal values.

6. Encourage increased mobility to reduce bone resorption. Ideally, the patient should be out of bed and up in a chair for at least 6 hours a day.

7. Avoid vitamin D preparations (see Table 9-1) because they increase intestinal absorption of calcium.

**Altered urinary elimination** related to dysuria, urgency, frequency, and polyuria secondary to administration of diuretics, calcium stone formation, or changes in renal function occurring with hypercalcemia.

Desired outcome: The patient exhibits voiding pattern and urine characteristics that are normal for the patient.

1. Monitor intake and output (I&O) hourly. Alert the physician to unusual changes in urine volume, for example, oliguria alternating with polyuria, which may signal urinary tract obstruction, or to continuous polyuria, which may be indicative of nephrogenic diabetes insipidus.

2. Because hypercalcemia can impair renal function, monitor the patient's renal function carefully: urine output, blood urea nitrogen (BUN), and creatinine.

3. Provide the patient with a low-calcium diet and avoid use of calcium-containing medications (e.g., antacids such as Tums).

4. Assess the patient for indicators of kidney stone formation: intermittent pain, nausea, vomiting, and hematuria. Encourage the intake of fruits (e.g., cranberries, prunes, or plums) that leave an acid ash in the urine. An acidic urine reduces the risk of calcium stone formation. Also, increase fluid intake (at least 3 L in unrestricted patients) to reduce the risk of renal stone formation.

5. Hypercalcemia leads to an increase in calcium in the urine, which inhibits the kidneys' ability to concentrate urine (nephrogenic diabetes inspidus). This leads to polyuria and potential volume depletion. Be alert to polyuria. Also, monitor for signs of volume depletion when giving diuretics: decreased BP, CVP, PAP; increased HR.

 ## Patient-Family Teaching Guidelines

Give the patient and significant others verbal and written instructions for the following:

1. Medications, including drug name, purpose, dosage, frequency, precautions, and potential side effects.
2. Signs and symptoms of hypercalcemia.
3. Foods and over-the-counter medications (e.g., antacids) that are high in calcium. See the box on p. 111 for a list of foods high in calcium content. Also, instruct patients to avoid vitamin supplements containing vitamins D and A.
4. If stone formation is a concern, encourage the intake of foods that leave an acid ash in the urine. Review signs and symptoms of nephrolithiasis.
5. After hospital discharge, it is important for the patient to increase fluid intake (up to 4 L in nonrestricted patients) to minimize risk of stone formation.
6. Importance of safe weight-bearing activities to decrease bone resorption.

# Disorders of Phosphorus Balance

**10**

Phosphorus is the primary anion of the intracellular fluid (ICF). Approximately 85% of the body's phosphorus is located in the bones and teeth, 14% is in the soft tissue, and less than 1% is within the extracellular fluid (ECF). Because of the large intracellular store, under certain acute conditions phosphorus may move into or out of the cell, causing dramatic changes in plasma phosphorus. Chronically, substantial increases or decreases can occur in intracellular phosphorus levels without significantly altering plasma levels. Thus plasma phosphorus levels do not necessarily reflect intracellular levels. Although most laboratories measure and report elemental phosphorus, nearly all the phosphorus in the body exists in the form of phosphate ($PO_4^{3-}$) and the terms phosphorus and phosphate often are used interchangeably.

Phosphorus is an important constituent of all body tissues and has a wide variety of vital functions, including formation of energy-storing substances (e.g., adenosine triphosphate [ATP]); formation of red blood cell 2,3-diphosphoglycerate (DPG), which facilitates oxygen delivery to the tissues; metabolism of carbohydrates, protein, and fat; and maintenance of acid-base balance. In addition, phosphorus is critical to normal nerve and muscle function and provides structural support to bones and teeth. Plasma $PO_4^{3-}$ levels vary with age, gender, and diet. Levels decrease with increasing age, with the exception of a slight rise in $PO_4^{3-}$ in women following menopause. Glucose, insulin, or sugar-containing foods cause a temporary drop in $PO_4^{3-}$ because of a shift of phosphorus into the cells.

Acid-base status also affects phosphorus balance. Alkalosis, particularly respiratory alkalosis, may cause hypophosphatemia as a result of an intracellular shift of phosphorus. The exact mechanism for this shift is not fully understood but may be related to an alkalosis-induced cellular glycolysis with increased formation of phosphorus-containing metabolic intermediates. Respiratory acidosis may cause a shift of phosphorus out of the cells and contribute to hyperphosphatemia.

The level of ECF phosphorus is regulated by a combination of factors, including dietary intake, intestinal absorption, renal excretion, and hormonally regulated bone resorption and deposition. Parathyroid hormone (PTH) secretion results in increased absorption of phosphorus from the gastrointestinal (GI) tract and increased movement of phosphorus out of the bone. However, PTH also increases urinary excretion of phosphorus. Phosphorus balance is closely tied to that of calcium. Normal range for serum phosphorus is 2.5 to 4.5 mg/dl (1.7 to 2.6 mEq/L).

# Hypophosphatemia

Hypophosphatemia (serum phosphorus <2.5 mg/dl) may be caused by transient intracellular shifts, increased urinary losses, decreased intestinal absorption, or increased cellular use (see "History and Risk Factors," in the following section). Severe phosphorus deficiency may also occur with alcoholism, especially during acute withdrawal, resulting from poor dietary intake, vomiting and diarrhea, hyperventilation, use of phosphorus-binding antacids, and increased urinary losses. In addition, a combination of factors may lead to hypophosphatemia in diabetic ketoacidosis (DKA). In DKA there is a significant loss of phosphorus in the urine secondary to the glucose-induced osmotic diuresis. This developing hypophosphatemia is masked, however, by the movement of phosphorus out of the cells as a result of increased tissue catabolism (cellular breakdown). When ketoacidosis is treated with glucose, insulin, and fluids, there is a dramatic shift of phosphorus back into the cells and the existing phosphorus depletion then becomes apparent. For more information about DKA, see Chapter 20.

## Assessment

1. **Clinical manifestations:** Patients may present with acute symptoms caused by sudden decreases in serum phosphorus, or symptoms may develop gradually, resulting from chronic phosphorus deficiency. The majority of symptoms are secondary to decreases in ATP and 2,3-DPG.

- *Acute:* Confusion, seizures, coma, chest pain resulting from poor oxygenation of the myocardium, muscle pain, increased susceptibility to infection, numbness and tingling of the fingers and circumoral region, and incoordination.
- *Chronic:* Memory loss, lethargy, and bone pain.

2. **Physical assessment:**
   - *Acute:* Decreased strength as evidenced by difficulty speaking, weakness of respiratory muscles, and weakening hand grasp. Hypoxemia may cause an increased respiratory rate (RR) and respiratory alkalosis (secondary to hyperventilation). NOTE: Respiratory alkalosis causes phosphorus to move intracellularly, aggravating the existing hypophosphatemia.
   - *Chronic:* Bruising and bleeding may occur because of platelet dysfunction. Lethargy, weakness, joint stiffness, arthralgia, osteomalacia, cyanosis, and pseudofractures may occur.

3. **Hemodynamic measurements:** Severely depleted patients may show signs of decreased myocardial function, including increased pulmonary artery wedge pressure (PAWP), decreased cardiac output (CO), and decreased blood pressure (BP) with decreased response to pressor agents.

4. **History and risk factors:**
   - *Intracellular shifts:* Carbohydrate load, respiratory alkalosis (see Chapter 14), nutritional recovery (usually associated with total parenteral nutrition [TPN]), androgen therapy, and recovery from burns.
   - *Increased use resulting from increased tissue repair:* TPN with inadequate phosphorus content; recovery from protein-calorie malnutrition.
   - *Increased urinary losses:* Hypomagnesemia (see Chapter 11), hypokalemia, hyperparathyroidism, use of thiazide diuretics, familial hypophosphatemic rickets, and Fanconi's syndrome.
   - *Reduced intestinal absorption or increased intestinal loss:* Use of phosphorus-binding antacids (e.g., aluminum hydroxide antacids such as Amphojel or Alternajel), vomiting and diarrhea, and malabsorption disorders such as vitamin D deficiency.

■ *Mixed causes:* Alcoholism, DKA (with treatment), and severe burns.

## Diagnostic Tests

1. **Serum phosphorus:** Will be less than 2.5 mg/dl (1.7 mEq/L).
   - ■ *Moderate hypophosphatemia:* 1 to 2.5 mg/dl.
   - ■ *Severe hypophosphatemia:* less than 1 mg/dl.
2. **PTH level:** Will be elevated in hyperparathyroidism.
3. **Serum magnesium:** May be decreased because of increased urinary excretion of magnesium in hypophosphatemia.
4. **Alkaline phosphatase:** Increased with increased osteoblastic activity.
5. **X-ray films:** May reveal skeletal changes of osteomalacia or rickets.

## Collaborative Management

1. **Identification and elimination of the cause:** For example, avoiding use of phosphorus-binding antacids (aluminum, magnesium, or calcium gels or antacids).
2. **Phosphorus supplementation:** Mild hypophosphatemia may be treated by increasing intake of high-phosphorus foods (see the box below). Mild to moderate hypophosphatemia usually can be treated with oral phosphate supplements such as Neutra Phos (sodium and potassium phosphate) or Phospho-Soda (sodium phosphate). Intravenous (IV) sodium phosphate or potassium phosphate is

### Foods High in Phosphorus

Meats, especially organ meats (e.g., brain, liver, kidney)
Fish
Poultry
Milk and milk products (e.g., cheese, ice cream, cottage cheese)
Whole grains (e.g., oatmeal, bran, barley)
Seeds (e.g., pumpkin, sesame, sunflower)
Nuts (e.g., Brazil, peanuts)
Eggs and egg products (e.g., eggnog, souffles)
Dried beans and peas

necessary in cases of severe hypophosphatemia or when the GI tract is nonfunctional.

## Nursing Diagnoses and Interventions

**Altered protection** related to sensory or neuromuscular dysfunction secondary to hypophosphatemia-induced central nervous system (CNS) disturbances.

**Desired outcome:** The patient verbalizes orientation to person, place, and time and does not exhibit evidence of injury caused by altered sensorium.

1. Monitor serum phosphorus levels in patients at increased risk. Notify the physician of decreased levels.
2. Apprehension, confusion, and paresthesias are signals of developing hypophosphatemia. Assess and document the level of consciousness (LOC), orientation, and neurologic status with each vital sign check. Reorient the patient as necessary. Alert the physician to significant changes.
3. Inform the patient and significant others that altered sensorium is temporary and will improve with treatment.
4. Do not administer IV phosphate at a rate greater than that recommended by the manufacturer. Potential complications of IV phosphorus administration include *tetany* resulting from hypocalcemia (serum calcium levels may drop suddenly if serum phosphorus levels increase suddenly [see pp. 107-108 for additional information]); *soft tissue calcification* (if the patient develops hyperphosphatemia, the calcium and phosphorus in the ECF may combine and form deposits in tissue [see p. 125]); and *hypotension,* caused by a too-rapid delivery. When IV phosphorus is administered as potassium phosphate, the infusion rate should not exceed 10 mEq/hr. Monitor the IV site for signs of infiltration because potassium phosphate can cause necrosis and sloughing of tissue (see pp. 97-99 for precautions when administering IV potassium).
5. Keep the side rails up and the bed in its lowest position, with wheels locked.
6. Use reality therapy such as clocks, calendars, and familiar objects. Keep these articles at the bedside, within the patient's visual field.
7. If the patient is at risk for seizures, pad the side rails and keep an airway at the bedside.

**Impaired gas exchange** related to altered oxygen-carrying capacity of the blood secondary to decreased 2,3-DPG and decreased gas exchange secondary to decreased strength of respiratory muscles. NOTE: With decreased 2,3-DPG levels, the oxyhemoglobin dissociation curve will shift to the right. That is, at a given oxygen tension of arterial blood ($Pao_2$) level, more oxygen will be bound to hemoglobin and less will be available to the tissues.

**Desired outcome:** The patient exhibits normal respiratory function as evidenced by RR 12 to 20 breaths/min with normal depth and pattern (eupnea); normal skin color; absence of chest pain; and orientation to person, place, and time.

1. Monitor rate and depth of respirations in patients who are severely hypophosphatemic. Alert the physician to changes.
2. Assess the patient for signs of hypoxemia: restlessness, confusion, increased RR, complaints of chest pain, and cyanosis (a late sign). Monitor arterial blood gas (ABG) values.
3. There is an increased incidence of hypophosphatemia in artificially ventilated patients. Monitor serum phosphate levels in these patients. Hypophosphatemia may contribute to difficulty in weaning patients from ventilators.
4. Administer phosphorus as prescribed.

**Impaired physical mobility** (or risk of same) related to osteomalacia with bone pain and fractures caused by movement of phosphorus out of the bone secondary to chronic hypophosphatemia; or muscle weakness and acute rhabdomyolysis (breakdown of striated muscle) secondary to severe hypophosphatemia.

**Desired outcome:** The patient has mobility without evidence of weakness, pain, or fractures.

1. Monitor all patients with suspected hypophosphatemia for evidence of decreasing muscle strength. Perform serial assessments of hand grasp strength and clarity of speech. Consult with the physician for changes.
2. Monitor serum phosphorus levels for evidence of worsening hypophosphatemia. Alert the physician to changes.
3. Assist the patient with ambulation and with activities of daily living. Keep personal items within easy reach.
4. Encourage the intake of foods high in phosphorus. See the box on p. 121.
5. Medicate the patient for pain as prescribed.

**Decreased cardiac output** related to negative inotropic changes associated with reduced myocardial functioning secondary to severe phosphorus depletion.

**Desired outcomes:** The patient's cardiac output is adequate as evidenced by central venous pressure (CVP) below 6 mm Hg, heart rate (HR) 100 or fewer beats per minute (bpm), BP within the patient's normal range, and absence of the clinical signs of heart failure or pulmonary edema. Critical care patients exhibit pulmonary artery pressure (PAP) 20-30/8-15 mm Hg.

1. Monitor the patient for signs of heart failure or pulmonary edema: crackles (rales), rhonchi, shortness of breath (SOB), decreased BP, increased HR, increased PAP, or increased CVP.
2. Prevent the patient from hyperventilating if possible because respiratory alkalosis will cause an increased movement of phosphorus into the cells.

**Risk for infection** related to impaired white blood cell (WBC) functioning secondary to reduced ATP.

**Desired outcome:** The patient is free of infection as evidenced by afebrile state and absence of erythema, swelling, warmth, and purulent drainage at invasive sites.

1. Monitor temperature and secretions every 4 hours for evidence of infection. Culture suspicious secretions as prescribed.
2. Use meticulous, aseptic technique when changing dressings or manipulating indwelling lines (e.g., TPN catheters, IV needles).
3. Provide oral hygiene and skin care at regular intervals. Intact skin and membranes are the body's first line of defense against infection.

 ## Patient-Family Teaching Guidelines

Give the patient and significant others verbal and written instructions for the following:

1. Medications, including drug name, purpose, dosage, frequency, precautions, and potential side effects.
2. Indicators of hypophosphatemia and hyperphosphatemia. Review the symptoms that necessitate immediate medical attention: weakness, SOB, and numbness and tingling of fingers and circumoral region. For patients at risk for chronic

hypophosphatemia, alert them to the need for notifying the physician of the presence of bone pain.
3. Foods that are high in phosphorus, if a high-phosphorus diet is encouraged (see the box on p. 121).
4. Importance of using phosphorus-binding antacids *only* as prescribed by the physician.

# Hyperphosphatemia

Hyperphosphatemia occurs most often in the presence of renal insufficiency because of the kidneys' decreased ability to excrete excess phosphorus. In addition to renal failure, other causes of hyperphosphatemia include excessive intake of phosphates, extracellular shifts (i.e., movement of phosphorus out of the cell and into the ECF), cellular destruction with concomitant release of intracellular phosphorus, and decreased urinary losses that are unrelated to decreased renal function. As serum phosphorus levels increase, serum calcium levels often drop, which may cause hypocalcemia to develop (see Chapter 9). Hypocalcemia is most likely to occur in sudden, severe hyperphosphatemia (e.g., after IV administration of phosphates) or when the patient already is prone to hypocalcemia (e.g., with chronic renal failure).

The primary complication of hyperphosphatemia is metastatic calcification (i.e., the precipitation of calcium phosphate in the soft tissue, joints, and arteries). Precipitation of calcium phosphate occurs when the calcium-phosphorus product (calcium × phosphorus) exceeds 70. Chronic hyperphosphatemia in the patient with chronic renal failure may contribute to the development of renal osteodystrophy.

## Assessment

1. **Clinical manifestations:** Anorexia, nausea, vomiting, muscle weakness, hyperreflexia, tetany, and tachycardia. NOTE: Usually, patients experience few symptoms with hyperphosphatemia. The majority of symptoms that do occur relate to the development of hypocalcemia or soft tissue (metastatic) calcifications. Indicators of metastatic calcification include oliguria, corneal haziness, conjunctivitis, irregular HR, and papular eruptions.
2. **Physical assessment:** See "Hypocalcemia," p. 108. In

addition, see "Clinical manifestations," p. 125, for indicators of metastatic calcifications.

3. **Electrocardiogram (ECG) changes:** See "Hypocalcemia," p. 108. Deposition of calcium phosphate in the heart may lead to dysrhythmias and conduction disturbances.

4. **History and risk factors:**
   - *Renal failure:* Acute and chronic.
   - *Increased intake:* Excessive administration of phosphorus supplements, vitamin D excess with increased GI absorption, and excessive use of phosphorus-containing laxatives or enemas (especially in children).
   - *Extracellular shift:* Respiratory acidosis and DKA (before treatment).
   - *Cellular destruction:* Neoplastic disease (e.g., leukemia and lymphoma) treated with cytotoxic agents, increased tissue catabolism (breakdown), and rhabdomyolysis (breakdown of striated muscle).
   - *Decreased urinary losses:* Hypoparathyroidism and volume depletion.

## Diagnostic Tests

1. **Serum phosphorus:** Will be greater than 4.5 mg/dl (2.6 mEq/L).
   NOTE: Improper handling of blood specimens may result in factitious (false) hyperphosphatemia because of hemolysis of blood cells.

2. **Serum calcium level:** Useful in assessing potential consequences of treatment and diagnosis of primary problem.

3. **X-ray films:** May show skeletal changes of osteodystrophy.

4. **Parathyroid hormone:** Level will be decreased in hypoparathyroidism.

5. **Blood urea nitrogen (BUN) and creatinine:** To assess renal function.

## Collaborative Management

1. **Identification and elimination of the cause** (e.g., correction of volume depletion).

2. **Use of aluminum, magnesium, or calcium gels or antacids:** To bind phosphorus in the gut, thus increasing GI elimination of phosphorus (Table 10-1). NOTE: Magnesium antacids are avoided in renal failure because of the risk of hyper-

**Table 10-1   Phosphorus binding agents**

| Agent | Trade Name | Dosage Form |
| --- | --- | --- |
| Aluminum carbonate | Basajel | Capsule |
| Aluminum hydroxide | Alternagel | Liquid |
| | Alucap | Capsule |
| | Amphojel | Liquid |
| | Dialume | Capsule |
| | Nephrox | Liquid |
| Calcium acetate | PhosLo | Tablet |
| | Phos-Ex | Tablet |
| Calcium carbonate | Caltrate | Tablet |
| | Os-cal | Tablet |
| | Titralac | Liquid |
| | Tums | Tablet |
| Sucralfate | Carafate | Liquid, tablet |

magnesemia. Calcium preparations are preferred in chronic renal failure because chronic use of aluminum preparations may contribute to the development of bone disease. Serum phosphorus levels may be allowed to remain slightly elevated (4.5 to 6 mg/dl) in chronic renal failure to ensure adequate levels of 2,3-DPG. This helps limit the effects of chronic anemia on oxygen delivery to the tissues.

3. **Diet low in phosphorus:** See the box on p. 121 for a list of foods that should be avoided or limited.
4. **Dialytic therapy:** May be necessary for acute, severe hyperphosphatemia accompanied by symptomatic hypocalcemia.

## Nursing Diagnoses and Interventions

*ndx*

**Knowledge deficit:** The purpose of phosphate binders and the importance of reducing GI absorption of phosphorus to control hyperphosphatemia and prevent long-term complications.

**Desired outcome:** The patient describes the potential complications of uncontrolled hyperphosphatemia and the ways in which they can be prevented. NOTE: Because symptoms of hyperphosphatemia may be minimal, the prevention of long-term complications relies primarily on adequate patient education.

1. Teach patients the purpose of phosphate binders. Stress the need to take binders as prescribed with or after meals to maximize effectiveness.

2. Prepare patients for the possibility of constipation secondary to binder use. Encourage the use of bulk-building supplements or stool softener if constipation occurs. Phosphate-containing laxatives and enemas must be avoided.

3. Phosphate binders are available in liquid or capsule form. Confer with the physician regarding an alternate form or brand for individuals who find binders unpalatable or difficult to take. Phosphate binders vary in their aluminum, magnesium, or calcium content, however, and one may not be exchanged for another without first ensuring that the patient is receiving the same amount of elemental aluminum, magnesium, or calcium.

4. Encourage the patient to avoid or limit foods high in phosphorus (see the box on p. 121).

**Altered protection** related to precipitation of calcium phosphate in the soft tissue (e.g., cornea, lungs, kidneys, gastric mucosa, heart, and blood vessels) and periarticular region of the large joints (e.g., hips, shoulders, and elbows) or development of hypocalcemic tetany.

**Desired outcomes:** The patient exhibits no evidence of metastatic calcification or hypocalcemia. The calcium-phosphorus product (calcium × phosphorus) remains less than 70 mg/dl.

1. Monitor serum phosphorus and calcium levels. Alert the physician to abnormal values. Remember that phosphorus values may be kept slightly higher (4.5 to 6 mg/dl) in chronic renal failure patients to ensure adequate levels of 2,3-DPG, thereby minimizing effects of chronic anemia on oxygen delivery to the tissues.

2. Avoid vitamin D products (see Table 9-1) and calcium supplements until the serum phosphorus level approaches normal.

3. Alert the physician to indicators of metastatic calcification: oliguria, corneal haziness, conjunctivitis, irregular HR, and papular eruptions.

4. Monitor the patient for evidence of increasing hypocalcemia: numbness and tingling of the fingers and circumoral region, hyperactive reflexes, and muscle cramps. Notify the physician promptly if these symptoms develop because they occur before overt tetany. In addition, alert the physician if the patient has positive Trousseau's or Chvostek's signs because they signal latent tetany (see p. 108 for a discussion of these

signs and Chapter 9 for additional information regarding treatment and prevention of hypocalcemia).

5. Because hyperphosphatemia can impair renal function, monitor the patient's renal function carefully: urine output, BUN, and creatinine. For additional information, see Chapter 22.

## Patient-Family Teaching Guidelines

Give the patient and significant others verbal and written instructions for the following:

1. Medications, including drug name, purpose, dosage, frequency, precautions, and potential side effects.

2. Indicators of hyperphosphatemia and hypocalcemia. Review the symptoms that require immediate medical attention: weakness, SOB, and numbness and tingling of fingers and circumoral region. Alert patients with chronic hyperphosphatemia to the necessity of notifying the physician if symptoms of metastatic calcification occur.

3. Foods that are high in phosphorus and thus must be avoided or limited (see the box on p. 121).

4. Importance of avoiding phosphorus-containing over-the-counter medications: certain laxatives, enemas, and multivitamin and mineral supplements. Instruct the patient and significant others to read labels for the words *phosphorus* and *phosphate*.

# Disorders of Magnesium Balance

# 11

Magnesium is the body's fourth most abundant cation, yet its measurement and evaluation often are overlooked. Of the body's magnesium, approximately 50% to 60% is located in bone and approximately 1% is located in the extracellular fluid (ECF). The remaining magnesium is contained within the cells, thereby constituting the second most abundant intracellular cation after potassium. Magnesium is regulated by a combination of factors, including vitamin D-controlled gastrointestinal (GI) absorption and renal excretion. Normally, only about 30% to 40% of dietary magnesium is absorbed. Renal excretion of magnesium changes to maintain magnesium balance and is affected by sodium and calcium excretion, ECF volume, and the presence of parathyroid hormone (PTH). Excretion is decreased with increased PTH, decreased excretion of sodium or calcium, and fluid volume deficit.

Because magnesium is a major intracellular ion, it plays a vital role in normal cellular function. Specifically, it activates enzymes involved in the metabolism of carbohydrates and protein and triggers the sodium-potassium pump, thus affecting intracellular potassium levels. Magnesium is also important in the transmission of neuromuscular activity, neural transmission within the central nervous system (CNS), and myocardial functioning.

Normal serum magnesium level is 1.5 to 2.5 mEq/L. Approximately one fourth to one third of the plasma magnesium is bound to protein, a small portion is combined with other substances (complexed), and the remaining portion is free or ionized. It is the free ionized magnesium that is physiologically important. As with calcium levels, magnesium levels should be evaluated in combination with serum albumin levels. Low serum albumin levels will decrease the total magnesium level, whereas the amount of free ionized magnesium may be unchanged. Magnesium may be used as a therapeutic agent in the treatment of pregnancy-induced hypertension, ischemic heart disease, dysrhythmias, or asthma. Normal range for serum magnesium is 1.5 to 2.5 mEq/L.

# Hypomagnesemia

Hypomagnesemia (serum magnesium level <1.5 mEq/L) usually occurs because of decreased GI absorption or increased urinary loss. It also may occur with excessive GI loss (e.g., vomiting, diarrhea) or with prolonged administration of magnesium-free parenteral fluids. Alcoholics (see "History and risk factors," below) and critical care patients are the two most common patient populations. Hypomagnesemia is usually associated with hypocalcemia and hypokalemia (see p. 132 for additional information). Symptoms of hypomagnesemia tend to develop once the serum magnesium level drops below 1 mEq/L.

## Assessment

1. **Clinical manifestations:** Apathy, leg cramps, insomnia, mood changes, hallucinations, confusion, anorexia, nausea, vomiting, and paresthesias.
2. **Physical assessment:** Increased reflexes, tremors, convulsions, tetany, and positive Chvostek's and Trousseau's signs (see p. 108) in part caused by accompanying hypocalcemia. The patient also may have tachycardia and hypertension.
3. **Hemodynamic measurements:** See "Hypocalcemia," p. 108 and "Hypokalemia," p. 96.
4. **History and risk factors:**
   - *Chronic alcoholism:* A common cause of hypomagnesemia resulting from a combination of poor dietary intake, decreased GI absorption, and increased urinary excretion secondary to ethanol effect.
   - *Malabsorption syndrome:* Caused by cancer, colitis, pancreatic insufficiency, and surgical resection of the GI tract.
   - *Increased GI loss:* Prolonged vomiting or gastric suction and prolonged diarrhea.
   - *Administration of low-magnesium or magnesium-free parenteral solutions.*
   - *Diabetic ketoacidosis or poorly controlled diabetes:* As a

result of movement of magnesium out of the cell and loss in the urine because of osmotic diuresis secondary to glucosuria.

- *Drugs that enhance urinary excretion:* Loop diuretics, amphotericin, gentamicin, cisplatin, digoxin, cyclosporine, and pentamidine.
- *Protein-calorie malnutrition.*
- *Cardiopulmonary bypass.*

## Diagnostic Tests

1. **Serum magnesium level:** Will be less than 1.5 mEq/L. Unfortunately, a normal serum magnesium level does not eliminate the possibility of an intracellular deficiency.
2. **Serum ionized magnesium level:** A new test that provides a better indicator of intracellular magnesium because intracellular and extracellular levels of ionized magnesium are similar.
3. **Urinary magnesium level:** Helps identify renal causes of magnesium depletion; may be performed after parenteral administration of magnesium sulfate (magnesium loading test).
4. **Serum albumin level:** A decreased albumin level may cause a decreased magnesium level because of a reduction in protein-bound magnesium. The amount of free ionized magnesium may be unchanged.
5. **Serum potassium level:** May be decreased because of failure of the cellular sodium-potassium pump to move potassium into the cell and the accompanying loss of potassium in the urine. This hypokalemia may be resistant to potassium replacement until the magnesium deficit has been corrected.
6. **Serum calcium level:** Hypomagnesemia may lead to hypocalcemia caused by a reduction in the release and action of PTH. PTH is the primary regulator of serum calcium levels (see Chapter 9).
7. **Electrocardiogram (ECG) evaluations:** May reflect magnesium, as well as calcium and potassium deficiencies: tachyarrhythmias, prolonged PR and QT intervals, widening of the QRS, ST-segment depression, and flattened T waves. Increased digitalis effect, as evidenced by multifocal or bigeminal premature ventricular contractions (PVCs), paroxysmal atrial tachycardia with varying atrioventricular

(AV) block, and other heart blocks, also may occur. Dysrhythmias associated with hypomagnesemia include ventricular ectopy, Torsades de pointes, and atrial fibrillation.

## Collaborative Management

1. **Identification and elimination of the cause:** For example, adequate replacement of magnesium in total parenteral nutrition (TPN) solutions.
2. **Intravenous (IV) or intramuscular (IM) magnesium sulfate (MgSO$_4$):** For severe or symptomatic hypomagnesemia.
3. **Oral magnesium:** Magnesium oxide (Mag-ox) or magnesium chloride (Slow-Mag) preparations may be used to treat mild or chronic hypomagnesemia. The dose is based on the amount of elemental magnesium contained in each preparation.
4. **Increased dietary intake of magnesium:** See the box below.

## Nursing Diagnoses and Interventions

**Altered protection** related to sensory or neuromuscular dysfunction secondary to hypomagnesemia.

**Desired outcomes:** The patient does not exhibit evidence of injury caused by complications of severe hypomagnesemia. Serum magnesium levels are within normal range (1.5 to 2.5 mEq/L).

1. Monitor serum magnesium levels in patients at risk for developing hypomagnesemia, for example, those who are

### Foods High in Magnesium

Green, leafy vegetables (e.g., beet greens, collard greens)
Seafood and meat
Nuts and seeds
Wheat bran
Soy flour
Legumes
Bananas
Oranges
Grapefruit
Chocolate
Molasses
Coconuts

alcohol abusers or receiving medications that increase urinary excretion. Alert the physician to abnormal values. NOTE: Symptomatic hypomagnesemia may be mistakenly attributed to delirium tremens of chronic alcoholism. Be especially alert to indicators of magnesium deficit in these patients.

2. Administer IV $MgSO_4$ with caution. Refer to manufacturer's guidelines. Too-rapid administration may lead to dangerous hypermagnesemia with cardiac or respiratory arrest. Patients receiving IV magnesium should be monitored for decreasing blood pressure (BP), labored respirations, and diminished patellar (knee jerk) reflex. An absent patellar reflex is a signal of hyporeflexia caused by dangerous hypermagnesemia. Should any of these changes occur, stop the infusion and notify the physician *stat* (see p. 138). Keep calcium gluconate at the bedside in the event of hypocalcemic tetany or sudden hypermagnesemia.

3. For patients with chronic hypomagnesemia, administer oral (PO) magnesium supplements as prescribed. All magnesium supplements should be given with caution in patients with reduced renal function because of an increased risk of the development of hypermagnesemia. Diarrhea is a common side effect of PO magnesium supplements. Consult with the physician if diarrhea develops.

4. Encourage the intake of foods high in magnesium in appropriate patients (see the box on p. 133). NOTE: For most patients, a regular diet usually is adequate.

5. Keep symptomatic patients on seizure precautions. Decrease environmental stimuli (e.g., keep the room quiet, use subdued lighting).

6. Caution patients in whom hypocalcemia is suspected against hyperventilation. Respiratory alkalosis may precipitate tetany because of increased calcium binding.

7. Dysphagia may occur in hypomagnesemia. Test the patient's ability to swallow water before giving food or medications.

8. Assess and document the level of consciousness (LOC), orientation, and neurologic status with each vital sign (VS) check. Reorient the patient as necessary. Consult the physician for significant changes. Inform the patient and

significant others that altered mood and sensorium are temporary and will improve with treatment.

9. Consult with the physician for patients who are receiving magnesium-free solutions (e.g., TPN) for prolonged periods.

10. See "Hypokalemia," pp. 96-102 and "Hypocalcemia," pp. 110-112, for nursing care of these disorders. NOTE: Because magnesium is necessary for the movement of potassium into the cell, intracellular potassium deficits cannot be corrected until hypomagnesemia has been treated.

**Decreased cardiac output** related to electrical alterations associated with tachyarrhythmias or digitalis toxicity secondary to hypomagnesemia.

**Desired outcome:** ECG shows normal configuration and the heart rate (HR) is within normal range for the patient.

1. Monitor HR and regularity with each VS check. Alert the physician to changes.

2. Assess the ECG in the patient on continuous ECG monitoring.

3. Because hypomagnesemia (and hypokalemia) potentiates the cardiac effects of digitalis, monitor patients taking digitalis for digitalis-induced dysrhythmias. ECG changes may include multifocal or bigeminal PVCs, paroxysmal atrial tachycardia with varying AV block, and other heart blocks. Monitor for pulse changes in the non-ECG monitored setting.

**Nutrition altered:** Less than body requirements of magnesium related to history of poor intake or anorexia, nausea, and vomiting secondary to hypomagnesemia.

**Desired outcome:** The patient verbalizes knowledge of foods high in magnesium content and demonstrates consumption of these foods during meals.

1. Encourage the intake of small, frequent meals.

2. Teach the patient about foods high in magnesium content (see the box on p. 133) and encourage the intake of these foods.

3. Medicate with antiemetics as prescribed.

4. Include the patient, significant others, and the dietitian in meal planning as appropriate.

5. Provide oral hygiene before meals to enhance appetite.

# Patient-Family Teaching Guidelines

Give the patient and significant others verbal and written instructions for the following:

1. Medications, including drug name, purpose, dosage, frequency, precautions, and potential side effects.
2. Indicators of hypomagnesemia, hypermagnesemia, and hypocalcemia. Emphasize the symptoms that necessitate immediate medical attention: numbness and tingling of fingers and circumoral region, muscle cramps, altered sensorium, and irregular or rapid pulse.
3. Foods that are high in magnesium (see the box on p. 133). Review the prescribed diet with the patient.
4. Referrals to Alcoholics Anonymous, Al-anon, and Al-a-teen as appropriate for the alcoholic patient and his or her significant others.

# Hypermagnesemia

Hypermagnesemia (serum magnesium level >2.5 mEq/L) occurs almost exclusively in individuals with renal failure who have an increased intake of magnesium (e.g., use of magnesium-containing medications). It also may occur in acute adrenocortical insufficiency (Addison's disease) or during hypothermia. In rare cases hypermagnesemia occurs because of excessive use of magnesium-containing medications (e.g., antacids, laxatives, enemas). The primary symptoms of hypermagnesemia are the result of depressed peripheral and central neuromuscular transmission. Symptoms usually do not occur until the magnesium level exceeds 4 mEq/L.

## Assessment

1. **Clinical manifestations:** Nausea, vomiting, flushing, diaphoresis, sensation of heat, altered mental functioning, drowsiness, coma, and muscular weakness or paralysis. Paralysis of the respiratory muscles may occur when the magnesium level exceeds 10 mEq/L.
2. **Physical assessment:** Hypotension, soft tissue (metastatic) calcification (see p. 125), bradycardia, and decreased deep tendon reflexes. The patellar (knee jerk) reflex is lost once the magnesium level exceeds 8 mEq/L.
3. **Hemodynamic measurements:** Decreased arterial pressure because of peripheral vasodilation.

4. **History and risk factors:**
   - *Decreased excretion of magnesium:* Renal failure or adrenocortical insufficiency.
   - *Increased intake of magnesium:* Excessive use of magnesium-containing antacids, enemas, and laxatives or excessive administration of magnesium sulfate (e.g., in the treatment of hypomagnesemia or pregnancy-induced hypertension).

## Diagnostic Tests

1. **Serum magnesium level:** Will exceed 2.5 mEq/L.
2. **ECG findings:** Prolonged QT interval and AV block may occur in severe hypermagnesemia (levels >12 mEq/L).

## Collaborative Management

1. **Removal of cause:** For example, discontinuing or avoiding use of magnesium-containing medications or supplements, especially in patients with decreased renal function. See the box below for a list of medications that contain magnesium.

---

### Magnesium-Containing Medications

**Antacids**

Aludrox
Camalox
Di-Gel
Gaviscon
Gelusil and Gelusil II
Maalox and Maalox Plus
Mylanta and Mylanta II
Riopan
Simeco
Tempo

**Magnesium-Containing Mineral Supplements**

**Laxatives**

Magnesium hydroxide (milk of magnesium, Haley's M-O)
Magnesium citrate
Magnesium sulfate (Epsom salts)

2. **Diuretics and 0.45% sodium chloride solution:** To enhance magnesium excretion in patients with adequate renal function.

3. **IV calcium gluconate, 10 ml of a 10% solution:** To antagonize the neuromuscular effects of magnesium for patients with potentially lethal hypermagnesemia.

4. **Dialysis with magnesium-free dialysate:** For patients with severely decreased renal function.

## Nursing Diagnoses and Interventions

**Altered protection** related to altered mental functioning, drowsiness and weakness, or metastatic calcification secondary to hypermagnesemia.

**Desired outcomes:** The patient verbalizes orientation to person, place, and time and does not exhibit evidence of injury caused by complications of hypermagnesemia. The patient is asymptomatic of soft tissue (metastatic) calcifications: oliguria, corneal haziness conjunctivitis, irregular HR, and papular eruptions. Serum magnesium levels are within normal range (1.5 to 2.5 mEq/L).

1. Monitor serum magnesium levels in patients at risk for developing hypermagnesemia, for example, those with chronic renal failure or women being treated for pregnancy-induced hypertension or preterm labor.

2. Assess and document LOC, orientation, and neurologic status (e.g., hand grasp) with each VS check. Assess patellar (knee jerk) reflex in patients with a moderately elevated magnesium level (>5 mEq/L). With the patient lying flat, support the knee in a moderately flexed position and tap the patellar tendon firmly just below the patella. Normally, the knee will extend. An absent reflex suggests a magnesium level of 7 mEq/L or higher. Consult with the physician for significant changes.

3. Reassure the patient and significant others that altered mental functioning and muscle strength will improve with treatment.

4. Keep the side rails up and the bed in its lowest position, with the wheels locked.

5. Assess the patient for the development of soft tissue calcification. Consult with the physician for significant findings.

6. Infants born to mothers receiving parenteral magnesium

should be monitored for hypermagnesemia (e.g., neurologic depression, low Apgar scores).

7. Hypermagnesemia is often treated with IV calcium because it reverses the toxic effects of excess magnesium. The effects are temporary and repeated doses may be necessary. Keep calcium at the bedside of symptomatic patients.

**Knowledge deficit:** Importance of avoiding excessive or inappropriate use of magnesium-containing medications, especially for patients with chronic renal failure.

Desired outcome: The patient verbalizes the importance of avoiding unusual magnesium intake and identifies potential sources of unwanted magnesium.

1. Caution patients with chronic renal failure to review all over-the-counter medications with the health care provider before use.

2. Provide a list of common magnesium-containing medications (see the box on p. 137).

3. Patients with renal failure usually are on vitamin supplements. Caution these patients to avoid combination vitamin-mineral supplements because they usually contain magnesium.

## Patient-Family Teaching Guidelines

Give the patient and significant others verbal and written instructions for the following:

1. Medications, including drug name, dosage, purpose, schedule, precautions, and potential side effects.

2. Indicators of hypermagnesemia. Review symptoms that require immediate medical attention: altered mental functioning, drowsiness, and muscle weakness.

3. Magnesium-containing medications that should be avoided (see the box on p. 137).

4. The need to avoid magnesium-containing mineral supplements.

# Overview of Acid-Base Balance

12

For optimal functioning of the cells, metabolic processes maintain a steady balance between acids and bases. Arterial pH is an indirect measurement of hydrogen ion ($H^+$) concentration (i.e., the greater the concentration, the more acidic the solution and the lower the pH; the lower the concentration, the more alkaline the solution and the higher the pH) and is a reflection of the balance between carbon dioxide ($CO_2$), which is regulated by the lungs, and bicarbonate ($HCO_3^-$), a base regulated by the kidneys. $CO_2$ dissolves in solution to form carbonic acid ($H_2CO_3$), which is the key acid component in acid-base balance. Because $H_2CO_3$ is difficult to measure directly and $CO_2$ and $H_2CO_3$ are in balance, the acid component is expressed as $CO_2$ instead of $H_2CO_3$.

Normal acid-base ratio is 1:20, representing one part $CO_2$ (potential $H_2CO_3$) to twenty parts $HCO_3^-$. If this balance is altered, derangements in pH occur: if extra acids are present or there is a loss of base and the pH is less than 7.40, acidosis exists; if extra base is present or there is loss of acid and the pH is greater than 7.40, alkalosis is present. Several mechanisms regulate acid-base balance. These mechanisms are exceptionally sensitive to minute changes in pH and the body usually is able to maintain pH without outside intervention, if not at a normal level, at least within a life-sustaining range.

## Buffer System Responses
### Buffers

Buffers are present in all body fluids and act immediately (within 1 second) after an abnormal pH occurs. They combine with excess acid or base to form substances that do not affect pH. Their effect, however, is limited.

1. **Bicarbonate:** The most important buffer, it is present in the largest quantity in body fluids. It is generated by the kidneys and aids in the excretion of $H^+$.
2. **Phosphate:** Aids in the excretion of $H^+$ in the renal tubules.
3. **Ammonium:** After an acid load, ammonia ($NH_3$) is produced by the renal tubular cell and is combined with $H^+$ in the renal tubule to form ammonium ($NH_4^+$). This process allows greater renal excretion of $H^+$.
4. **Protein:** Present in cells, blood, and plasma. Hemoglobin is the most important protein buffer.

## Respiratory System

Hydrogen ions exert direct action on the respiratory center in the brain. Acidemia increases alveolar ventilation to 4 to 5 times the normal level, whereas alkalemia decreases alveolar ventilation to 50% to 75% of the normal level. The response occurs quickly—within 1 to 2 minutes—during which time the lungs eliminate or retain $CO_2$ in direct relation to arterial pH. Although the respiratory system cannot correct imbalances completely with healthy lungs, it is 50% to 70% effective.

## Renal System

The renal system regulates acid-base balance by increasing or decreasing $HCO_3^-$ concentration in body fluids. This is accomplished through a series of complex reactions that involve $H^+$, sodium ion ($Na^+$), and $HCO_3^-$ secretion, reabsorption, and conservation, and $NH_3$ synthesis for excretion in the urine. $H^+$ secretion is regulated by the amount of $CO_2$ in extracellular fluid (ECF): the greater the concentration of $CO_2$, the greater the amount of $H^+$ secretion, resulting in an acidic urine. When $H^+$ is excreted, $HCO_3^-$ is generated by the kidneys, helping maintain the 1:20 balance of acids and bases. When ECF is alkalotic, the kidneys conserve $H^+$ and eliminate sodium bicarbonate, resulting in alkalotic urine. Although the kidneys' response to an abnormal pH is slow (several hours to days), healthy kidneys are usually able to adjust the imbalance to normal or near normal because of their ability to excrete large quantities of excess $HCO_3^-$ and $H^+$ from the body.

# Blood Gas Values

Blood gas analysis usually is based on arterial sampling. Venous values are given as a reference (Table 12-1).

## Arterial Blood Gas Analysis

ABG measurement is the best means of evaluating acid-base balance.

1. **pH:** Measures $H^+$ concentration to reflect acid-base status of the blood. Values reflect whether arterial pH is normal (7.40), acidic (<7.40), or alkalotic (>7.40). Because of the ability of compensatory mechanisms to "normalize" the pH, a near-normal value does not exclude the possibility of an acid-base disturbance.

2. **Paco$_2$:** Partial pressure of carbon dioxide in arterial blood. It is the respiratory component of acid-base regulation and is adjusted by changes in the rate and depth of pulmonary ventilation. Hypercapnia (Paco$_2$ >45 mm Hg) indicates alveolar hypoventilation and respiratory acidosis. Hyper-ventilation results in a Paco$_2$ less than 35 mm Hg and respiratory alkalosis in healthy lungs. Respiratory compensation occurs rapidly in metabolic acid-base disturbances. If any abnormality in Paco$_2$ exists, it is important to analyze pH and $HCO_3^-$ parameters to determine if the alteration in Paco$_2$ is the result of a primary respiratory disturbance or a compensatory response to a metabolic acid-base abnormality.

3. **Pao$_2$:** Partial pressure of oxygen in arterial blood. It has no primary role in acid-base regulation if it is within normal limits. The presence of hypoxemia with a Pao$_2$ less than 60 mm Hg can lead to anaerobic metabolism, resulting in lactic acid production and metabolic acidosis. There is a normal decline in Pao$_2$ in the elderly. Hypoxemia also may cause hyperventilation, resulting in respiratory alkalosis.

4. **Saturation:** Measures the degree to which hemoglobin is saturated by oxygen ($O_2$). It can be affected by changes in temperature, pH, and Paco$_2$. When the Pao$_2$ falls below 60 mm Hg, there is a large drop in saturation.

5. **Base excess or deficit:** Indicates, in general terms, the amount of blood buffer (hemoglobin and plasma bicarbonate) present. Abnormally high values reflect alkalosis; low values reflect acidosis. Normal value is ± 2.

**Table 12-1  Mixed venous blood gas values**

| | Arterial Values | | Mixed Venous Values | |
| --- | --- | --- | --- | --- |
| | Perfect | Range | | |
| pH | 7.40 | 7.35-7.45 | pH | 7.33-7.43 |
| $Paco_2$ | 40 mm Hg | 35-45 mm Hg | $Pco_2$ | 41-51 mm Hg |
| $Pao_2$ | 95 mm Hg | 80-95 mm Hg | $Po_2$ | 35-49 mm Hg |
| Saturation | 95%-99% | | Saturation | 70%-75% |
| Base excess | ±2 | | | |
| *Serum $HCO_3^-$ | 24 mEq/L | 22-26 mEq/L | $HCO_3^-$ | 24-28 mEq/L |

*Although serum bicarbonate is a buffer, it is usually reported as total $CO_2$ or $CO_2$ content and not as serum $HCO_3^-$. The serum $HCO_3^-$ concentration is usually obtained separately from the arterial blood gas (ABG) analysis and is critical in the determination of acid-base status. (The $HCO_3^-$ reported with ABG results is usually calculated from pH and $Paco_2$.) Serum $HCO_3^-$ values should be obtained with the initial ABG assessment and daily thereafter.) $Paco_2$, Partial pressure of carbon dioxide in arterial blood; $Pao_2$, partial pressure of oxygen in arterial blood; $HCO_3^-$, bicarbonate ion; $Pco_2$, partial pressure of carbon dioxide; $Po_2$, partial pressure of oxygen.

6. $HCO_3^-$: Serum bicarbonate is the major renal component of acid-base regulation. (It is reported as $CO_2$ content or total $CO_2$.) It is excreted or regenerated by the kidneys to maintain a normal acid-base environment. Decreased bicarbonate levels (<24 mEq/L) are indicative of metabolic acidosis (seen infrequently as a compensatory mechanism for respiratory alkalosis); elevated bicarbonate levels (>28 mEq/L) reflect metabolic alkalosis—either as a primary metabolic disorder or as a compensatory alteration in response to respiratory acidosis.

## Step-by-Step Guide to Arterial Blood Gas Analysis

A systematic step-by-step analysis critical to the accurate interpretation of ABG values. For further information, see Tables 12-2, 12-3, and 12-4.

1. **Step one:** Determine if pH is normal. If it deviates from 7.40, note how much it deviates and in which direction. For example, pH higher than 7.40 indicates alkalosis; pH less than 7.40 indicates acidosis. Is the pH in the normal range of 7.35 to 7.45 or is it in the critical range of greater than 7.55 or less than 7.20?

2. **Step two:** Check the $Paco_2$. If it deviates from 40 mm Hg, how much does it deviate and in which direction? Does the change in $Paco_2$ correspond to the direction of the change in pH? The pH and $Paco_2$ should move in opposite directions. For example, as the $Paco_2$ increases, the pH should decrease (acidosis); and as the $Paco_2$ decreases, the pH should increase (alkalosis).

3. **Step three:** Determine the $HCO_3^-$ value (may be referred to as $CO_2$ content or total $CO_2$). If it deviates from 24 mEq/L, note the degree and direction of deviation. Does the change in $HCO_3^-$ correspond to the change in pH? The $HCO_3^-$ and pH should move in the same direction. For example, if the $HCO_3^-$ decreases, the pH should decrease (acidosis); and as the $HCO_3^-$ increases, the pH should increase (alkalosis).

4. **Step four:** If both the $Paco_2$ and $HCO_3^-$ are abnormal, which value corresponds more closely to the pH value? For example, if the pH reflects acidosis, which value also reflects acidosis (an increased $Paco_2$ or a decreased $HCO_3^-$)? The

**Table 12-2    Arterial blood gas comparisons of acid-base disorders**

| | | Alkalosis | | | Acidosis | | |
|---|---|---|---|---|---|---|---|
| | | $Paco_2$ | pH | $HCO_3^-$ | $Paco_2$ | pH | $HCO_3^-$ |
| Simple | Respiratory | 25 | *7.60 | 24 | 50 | *7.15 | 25 |
| | Metabolic | 44 | 7.54 | 36 | 38 | 7.20 | 15 |
| Compensated | Respiratory | 25 | 7.54 | 21 | 66 | 7.37 | 34 |
| | Metabolic | 50 | 7.42 | 31 | 23 | 7.28 | 9 |
| Mixed disorder | | 40 | 7.56 | 38 | 50 | 7.20 | 20 |

*Note the greater changes in pH with acute respiratory disorders owing to delayed renal compensation.
$Paco_2$, Partial pressure of carbon dioxide in arterial blood; $HCO_3^-$, bicarbonate ion.

**Table 12-3**    Quick assessment guide to acid-base imbalances

| Acid-Base Imbalance | pH | $Pa_{CO_2}$ | $HCO_3^-$ |
|---|---|---|---|
| Acute respiratory acidosis | Decreased | Increased | No change |
| Chronic respiratory acidosis (compensated) | Decreased | Increased | Increased* |
| Acute respiratory alkalosis | Increased | Decreased | No change (a decrease will occur if condition has been present for hours, providing that renal function is adequate) |
| Chronic respiratory alkalosis | Increased | Decreased | Decreased* |
| Acute metabolic acidosis | Decreased | Decreased* | Decreased |

*Compensatory response.
$Pa_{CO_2}$, Partial pressure of carbon dioxide in arterial blood; $HCO_3^-$, bicarbonate ion;

| Clinical Signs and Symptoms | Common Causes |
| --- | --- |
| Tachycardia, tachypnea, diaphoresis, headache, restlessness leading to lethargy and coma, cyanosis, dysrhythmias, hypotension | Acute respiratory failure, cardiopulmonary disease, drug overdose, chest wall trauma, asphyxiation, CNS trauma/lesions, impaired muscles of respiration |
| Dyspnea and tachypnea, with increase in $CO_2$ retention that exceeds compensatory ability; progression to lethargy, confusion, and coma | COPD, extreme obesity (Pickwickian syndrome), superimposed infection on COPD |
| Paresthesias, especially of the fingers; dizziness | Hyperventilation, salicylate poisoning, hypoxemia (e.g., with pneumonia, pulmonary edema, pulmonary thromboembolism), gram-negative sepsis, CNS lesion, decreased lung compliance, inappropriate mechanical ventilation |
| No symptoms | Hepatic failure, CNS lesion, pregnancy |
| Tachypnea leading to Kussmaul respirations, hypotension, cold and clammy skin, coma, and dysrhythmias | Shock, cardiopulmonary arrest (with resultant lactic acid production), ketoacidosis (e.g., diabetes, starvation, alcohol abuse), acute renal failure, ingestion of acids (e.g., salicylates), diarrhea |

*CNS,* central nervous system; *COPD,* chronic obstructive pulmonary disease.

*Continued*

Table 12-3   Quick assessment guide to acid-base imbalances—cont'd

| Acid-Base Imbalance | pH | Paco$_2$ | HCO$_3^-$ |
|---|---|---|---|
| Chronic metabolic acidosis | Decreased | Decreased* (not as much as acute metabolic acidosis) | Decreased |
| Acute metabolic alkalosis | Increased | Increased* (can be as great as 60) | Increased |
| Chronic metabolic alkalosis | Increased | Increased* | Increased |

*Compensatory response.

value that more closely corresponds to the pH and deviates more from normal points to the primary disturbance responsible for the alteration in pH. A mixed metabolic-respiratory disturbance or compensatory elements may be present when both HCO$_3^-$ and Paco$_2$ are abnormal.

5. **Step five:** Check Pao$_2$ and O$_2$ saturation to determine whether they are decreased, normal, or increased. Decreased Pao$_2$ and O$_2$ saturation can lead to lactic acidosis and may signal the need for increased concentrations of O$_2$. Conversely, high Pao$_2$ may be indicative of the need to decrease delivered concentrations of O$_2$.

| Clinical Signs and Symptoms | Common Causes |
|---|---|
| Fatigue, anorexia, malaise (may be related to chronic disease process as well as acidosis) | Chronic renal failure |
| Muscular weakness and hyporeflexia (caused by severe hypokalemia), dysrhythmias, apathy, confusion, and stupor | Volume depletion ($Cl^-$ depletion) as a result of vomiting, gastric drainage, diuretic use, posthypercapnia; hyperadrenocorticism (e.g., Cushing's syndrome), aldosteronism, severe potassium depletion, excessive alkali intake |
| Usually asymptomatic | Upper GI losses through continuous drainage; correction of hypercapnia if $Na^+$ and $K^+$ depletion remains uncorrected |

$Cl^-$, Chloride ion; *GI,* gastrointestinal; *Na$^+$,* sodium ion; *K$^+$,* potassium ion.

## Mixed venous blood gases

Mixed venous gases are usually obtained from a pulmonary artery catheter. (Blood from a central venous line may also be used if a pulmonary catheter is not present.) Mixed venous gases reflect acid-base status and oxygenation at the tissue level, thus providing information about metabolic and circulatory functioning. ABGs give information about ventilatory function only.

## Arterial-Venous Difference

The difference between arterial $O_2$ content and venous $O_2$ content reflects the tissue extraction of $O_2$ (oxygen content is determined from $O_2$ saturation and hemoglobin). The normal

**Table 12-4**   Acid-base rules: general guidelines

| Disturbance | Change in pH | Compensatory Response* | Results of Compensation |
|---|---|---|---|
| **Respiratory Acidosis** | | | |
| Acute | pH $\downarrow$ 0.08 for every 10 mm Hg $\uparrow$ in $Paco_2$ | Immediate release of tissue buffers (i.e., $HCO_3^-$) | 1 mEq/L $\uparrow$ in $HCO_3^-$ from the patient's baseline for every 10 mm Hg $\uparrow$ in $Paco_2$ |
| Chronic | Depends on renal compensation; often near normal | $\uparrow$ Renal reabsorption of $HCO_3^-$; clinically evident after 8 hours; maximal effect 3-5 days | 3.5 mEq/L $\uparrow$ in $HCO_3^-$, for every 10 mm Hg $\uparrow$ in $Paco_2$ |
| **Respiratory Alkalosis** | | | |
| Acute | pH $\uparrow$ 0.08 for every 10 mm Hg $\downarrow$ in $Paco_2$ | Immediate release of tissue buffers | 2 mEq/L $\downarrow$ in $HCO_3^-$ from the patient's baseline for every 10 mm Hg $\downarrow$ in $Paco_2$ |
| Chronic | pH can be returned to normal if renal function is adequate | $\downarrow$ Renal reabsorption of $HCO_3^-$ | Maximal renal compensation causes $HCO_3^-$; to $\downarrow$ 5 mEq/L for every 10 mm Hg $\downarrow$ in $Paco_2$. Maximal effect can take 7-9 days and may *normalize pH* |

| | | | |
|---|---|---|---|
| **Metabolic Acidosis** | | | |
| Acute | pH ↓ 0.15 for every 10 mEq/L ↓ in $HCO_3^-$ | Hyperventilation occurs immediately | 1.2 mm Hg ↓ in $Paco_2$ for every 1 mEq/L ↓ in $HCO_3^-$ |
| Chronic | pH same as it would be if no respiratory compensation were present | Hyperventilation | The effects of hyperventilation last only a few days because the ↓ in $Paco_2$ causes a further ↓ in renal reabsorption of $HCO_3^-$ |
| **Metabolic Alkalosis** | | | |
| Acute | pH ↑ 0.15 for every 10 mEq/L ↑ in $HCO_3^-$ | Hypoventilation occurs immediately | 0.7 mm Hg ↑ in $Paco_2$ for every 1 mEq/L ↑ in $HCO_3^-$ |
| Chronic | pH same as it would be if respiratory compensation were present | Hypoventilation | The effects of hypoventilation last for only a few days because the ↑ in $Paco_2$ causes ↑ renal excretion of $H^+$ and ↑ serum $HCO_3^-$ |

*Compensatory responses in *healthy* lungs and kidneys.

$Paco_2$, Partial pressure of carbon dioxide in arterial blood; $HCO_3^-$, bicarbonate ion.

value for arterial $O_2$ content is 18 ml/100 ml of blood, whereas the normal value for venous blood or pulmonary artery $O_2$ content is 14 ml/100 ml of blood. The difference between these two values increases when ventricular performance is impaired, for example, right ventricular failure associated with congestive heart failure.

# Respiratory Acidosis

13

## Acute Respiratory Acidosis

Respiratory acidosis occurs secondary to alveolar hypoventilation and results in a carbon dioxide ($CO_2$) tension of arterial blood ($Paco_2$) greater than 40 mm Hg (hypercapnia) and a pH less than 7.40. $Paco_2$ derangements are direct reflections of the degree of ventilatory dysfunction. Normally, $CO_2$ excretion equals $CO_2$ production. When there is an excess accumulation of $CO_2$, the lungs are failing to eliminate the necessary amounts to maintain the $Paco_2$ at 40 mm Hg. The degree to which the increased $Paco_2$ alters the pH depends on both the rapidity of onset and the body's ability to compensate through the blood buffer and renal systems. Although the blood buffer system acts immediately, it usually is not sufficient to maintain a normal pH in the presence of an elevated $Paco_2$. There is a delay (hours to days) before the effects of renal compensation can be noted, therefore acute respiratory acidosis can have a profound impact on pH.

## Assessment

1. **Clinical manifestations:** Dyspnea; asterixis; restlessness leading to lethargy, confusion, and coma.
2. **Physical assessment:** Increased heart rate (HR) and respiratory rate (RR), diaphoresis, and cyanosis. Severe hypercapnia may cause cerebral vasodilation, resulting in increased intracranial pressure (ICP) with papilledema. Another finding may be dilated conjunctival and facial blood vessels.
3. **Monitoring parameters:** Presence of ventricular dysrhythmias and increased ICP.
4. **History and risk factors:** See also the box on p. 154.
   - *Acute respiratory disease:* Acute respiratory failure from a number of causes, including pneumonia, adult respi-

153

## Potential Causes of Acute Respiratory Acidosis

**Pulmonary/Thoracic Disorders**

Severe pneumonia
ARDS
Flail chest
Pneumothorax
Hemothorax
Smoke inhalation

**Increased Resistance to Air Flow**

Upper airway obstruction
Aspiration
Laryngospasm (anaphylaxis, severe hypocalcemia)
Severe bronchospasm
Severe, prolonged acute asthma attack

**CNS Depression**

Sedative overdose
Anesthesia
Cerebral trauma
Cerebral infarct

**Metabolic Causes**

High-carbohydrate diet

**Neuromuscular Abnormalities**

Guillain-Barré syndrome
Myasthenia gravis crisis
Hypokalemia
High-cervical cordotomy
Drugs (e.g., curare, aminoglycosides)
Toxins
Hypophosphatemia

**Systemic Causes**

Cardiac arrest
Massive pulmonary embolus
Severe pulmonary edema

**Mechanical Ventilation**

Fixed minute ventilation with increased $CO_2$ production
Inappropriate dead space
Equipment failure

*ARDS,* Adult respiratory distress syndrome; *CNS,* central nervous system; $CO_2$, carbon dioxide.

ratory distress syndrome (ARDS), and acute exacerbation of underlying pulmonary dysfunction.

- *Overdose of drugs:* Oversedation with drugs that cause respiratory center depression.
- *Chest wall trauma:* Flail chest and pneumothorax.
- *Central nervous-system trauma/lesions:* Can lead to depression of respiratory center.
- *Asphyxiation:* Mechanical obstruction and anaphylaxis.
- *Impaired respiratory muscles:* Can occur with hypokale-

mia, Guillain-Barré syndrome, and myasthenia gravis crisis.

- *Iatrogenic:* Inappropriate mechanical ventilation (increased dead space, insufficient rate or volume); high fraction of inspired oxygen ($Fio_2$) in the presence of chronic $CO_2$ retention.

## Diagnostic Tests

1. **Arterial blood gas (ABG) analysis:** Aids in diagnosis and determination of severity of respiratory acidosis. $Paco_2$ will be greater than 40 mm Hg and pH will be less than 7.40. All individuals with elevated $Paco_2$ will have some degree of hypoxemia while breathing room air. The hypoxemia is usually present first and is initially more pronounced than the hypercapnia. A small increase in $Paco_2$ indicates severe pulmonary dysfunction.
2. **Total $CO_2$:** Reflects metabolic and base balance. Initially, bicarbonate ion ($HCO_3^-$) values will be normal (24 to 28 mEq/L) unless a mixed disorder is present.
3. **Serum electrolytes:** Usually not altered, depending on etiology of respiratory acidosis.
4. **Chest x-ray:** Determines presence of underlying respiratory disease.
5. **Drug screen:** Determines presence and quantity of drug if an overdose is suspected.

## Collaborative Management

1. **Restoration of normal acid-base balance:** Accomplished by supporting respiratory function. If $Paco_2$ is greater than 50 to 60 mm Hg and clinical signs such as cyanosis and lethargy are present, the patient usually requires intubation and mechanical ventilation. Generally, use of sodium bicarbonate ($NaHCO_3$) is avoided because of the risk of metabolic alkalosis when the respiratory disturbance has been corrected. In patients with severe acidemia (pH <7.15), small doses of $NaHCO_3$ (44 to 88 mEq) may be given over 5 to 10 minutes. ($NaHCO_3$ should be avoided in patients with pulmonary edema.) Although a life-threatening pH must be corrected promptly to an acceptable level, a normal pH is not the immediate goal.
2. **Treatment of the underlying disorder.**

## Nursing Diagnoses and Interventions

**Impaired gas exchange** related to alveolar hypoventilation secondary to underlying disease process.

**Desired outcome:** The patient has adequate oxygen supply and alveolar ventilation as evidenced by oxygen tension of arterial blood ($Pa_{O_2}$) 60 mm Hg or higher, $Pa_{CO_2}$ 45 mm Hg or lower, pH 7.35 to 7.45, RR 12 to 20 breaths/min with a normal pattern and depth (eupnea), absence of adventitious breath sounds, and impairment of mental status and restlessness are reduced or absent.

1. Monitor serial ABG results to detect continued presence of hypercapnia or hypoxemia. Report significant findings (i.e., variances of 10 to 20 mm Hg in $Pa_{CO_2}$ or $Pa_{O_2}$).
2. Assess and document the character of respiratory effort: rate, depth, rhythm, and use of accessory muscles of respiration.
3. Assess the patient for signs and symptoms of respiratory distress: restlessness, anxiety, confusion, and tachypnea (RR >20 breaths/min).
4. Position the patient for comfort and to ensure optimal gas exchange. Usually, semi-Fowler's position allows for adequate expansion of the chest wall, but the specific pathologic process must be considered when positioning patients.
   - For unilateral lung disease in the patient who is ventilated mechanically, a side-lying (lateral decubitus) position may increase perfusion in the dependent (healthy) lung and increase ventilation to the upper (diseased) lung ("good side down" position).
   - For patients with ARDS requiring mechanical ventilation, the prone position may improve gas exchange by decreasing the edema and increasing the ventilation to the dependent lung area. Hypoventilation can occur in dependent areas with mechanical ventilation, resulting in atelectasis. Not all patients with ARDS will benefit from the prone position, and a brief trial (30 minutes) in this position is recommended to identify patients who can benefit from it. Improved ventilatory status will be noted by improvement in breath sounds and ABG values (increased $Pa_{CO_2}$ on the same oxygen concentration and ventilator settings).
5. Remove secretions by coughing or suctioning.

6. If ordered, monitor mechanical ventilation: ventilator settings, endotracheal and tracheal tube function, and ventilator and breathing circuit function.

**Sensory-perceptual alterations** related to disturbance in acid-base regulation.

**Desired outcome:** The patient verbalizes orientation to person, place, and time and does not exhibit evidence of injury caused by altered sensorium.

1. Monitor ABG and serum $CO_2$ results. Notify the physician regarding abnormal values and significant changes (i.e., variances of 10 to 20 mm Hg in $Paco_2$ and $Pao_2$). At frequent intervals assess and document the patient's level of consciousness (LOC) and orientation to person, place, and time.

2. Use reality therapy such as familiar photos, a calendar, and a clock with a face that is large enough for the patient to see. Keep these items at the bedside and within the patient's visual field.

3. Keep the bed in its lowest position, with all side rails up and the wheels locked.

4. If the patient is allowed out of bed, remind him or her to ask for assistance before getting up.

5. Offer confused patients the opportunity to toilet at frequent intervals. Many falls result from disoriented or unsteady patients' attempts to toilet.

6. Use a night light to minimize confusion in an unfamiliar and unlit environment.

7. If the patient's confusion persists despite reorientation, increase the frequency of observations, with concomitant reorientation and documentation. Alert the physician to continued or increasing confusion.

8. Reassure the patient and significant others that the patient's confusion will abate with treatment.

9. If the patient remains at risk for injury, obtain a prescription for a protective restraining device per agency policy.
   - Document the need for a restraining device based on the patient's behavior upon initiation and every 8 hours thereafter.
   - Choose the least restrictive device that will protect the patient. Add additional device(s) as needed, based on documented patient behaviors.

- Document the type of device used. A protective vest is applied to the upper torso with the crisscross or "V" in the front. Soft limb protectors are applied to the upper extremities (may be applied to upper and lower extremities in some cases).
- Monitor the patient every 15 to 30 minutes while restraints are in use, documenting mental status and response to protective device(s).
- Document the frequency (at least every 2 hours) of device removal, repositioning of patient, and reapplication of the device.

**Altered oral mucous membrane** related to abnormal breathing pattern.

Desired outcome: Absence of oral inflammation and infection.

1. Assess the patient's oral mucous membrane, lips, and tongue every 2 hours, noting presence of dryness, exudate, swelling, blisters, and ulcers.
2. If the patient is alert and able to take fluids orally, offer frequent sips of water or ice chips to alleviate dryness.
3. Perform mouth care every 2 to 4 hours, using a soft-bristled toothbrush to cleanse the teeth and a moistened cloth or toothette (small sponge on a stick) to moisten crusty areas or exudate on the tongue and oral mucosa. If the patient is intubated, suction the mouth to remove fluid and debris.
4. If indicated, use an artificial saliva preparation to assist in keeping the mucous membrane moist. Avoid use of lemon and glycerine swabs, which can contribute to dryness.
5. Apply vitamin A and D ointment in a lanolin-petrolatum base lip balm to keep lips from drying and to aid in healing cracked lips.

**Sleep pattern disturbance** related to frequent treatments and procedures.

Desired outcome: The patient sleeps undisturbed for at least 90 minutes at a time and relates a feeling of well being.

1. Gather information about the patient's normal sleep habits: bedtime rituals; usual position; hours of sleep required; number of pillows used; and sensitivity to light, noise, and touch. Based on data gathered, attempt to incorporate the patient's needs into his or her care plan.

# Laboratory Quick Reference Guide

## Tests to Evaluate Fluid Status

| Test | Value |
|---|---|
| Serum osmolality | 280-300 mOsm/kg |
| Hematocrit | 40%-54% (males), 37%-47% (females) |
| Blood urea nitrogen | 6-20 mg/dl |
| Urine osmolality | Physiologic range 50-1400 mOsm/kg, typical 300-900 mOsm/kg |
| Urine specific gravity | Physiologic range 1.001-1.040 Random specimen with normal fluid intake 1.010-1.020 |
| Urine sodium | Random specimen normal range 50-130 mEq/L |

---------------------------- FOLD HERE ----------------------------

## Related Tests

| Test | Value |
|---|---|
| Creatinine | 0.6-1.5 mg/dl |
| Serum albumin | 3.5-5.5 g/dl |

## Tests to Evaluate Electrolyte Balance

| Test | Reference value |
|---|---|
| Sodium | 135-145 mEq/L |
| Chloride | 95-108 mEq/L |
| Potassium | 3.5-5 mEq/L |
| Total $CO_2$ | 22-28 mEq/L |
| Calcium | 8.5-10.5 mg/dl |
|  | 4.3-5.3 mEq/L |
| Magnesium | 1.8-3 mg/dl |
|  | 1.5-2.5 mEq/L |
| Phosphorus | 2.5-4.5 mg/dl |
|  | 1.7-2.6 mEq/L |

## Tests to Evaluate Acid-Base Balance

### Arterial blood gases

| Test | Reference value |
|---|---|
| pH | 7.35-7.45 |
| $Paco_2$ | 35-45 mm Hg |
| $Pao_2$ | 80-95 mm Hg |
| $O_2$ saturation | 95%-99% |
| $HCO_3^-$ | 22-26 mEq/L |

### Other tests

| Test | Reference value |
|---|---|
| $CO_2$ content or total $CO_2$ | 22-28 mEq/L |
| Anion gap | 12 (± 2) mEq/L |
| Urine pH | Random speci-men 4.6-8 |
| Lactic acid | 0.5-1.6 mEq/L (arterial), 1.5-2.2 mEq/L (venous) |

2. Cluster activities and procedure to minimize need for interrupting the patient's sleep. Even brief (30-second) interruptions of sleep can result in feelings of fatigue.

3. Attempt to administer unpleasant or uncomfortable procedures or treatments at least 1 hour before bedtime to allow time for relaxation before the patient attempts to go to sleep.

4. Offer backrubs, repositioning, and relaxation techniques (quiet music, instructions for imagery) at bedtime.

5. If the patient requires a daytime nap because of fatigue, provide opportunities to sleep between 1 PM and 3 PM. Sleep attained at this time is most restful and least likely to disrupt night-time sleep. Discourage napping after 7 PM, as it may prevent the patient from falling asleep and maintaining a normal sleep cycle.

6. Monitor the level of daytime alertness and daytime functioning.

**Ineffective family coping** related to stress reaction secondary to catastrophic illness of family member.

**Desired outcome:** Family members exhibit improved coping mechanisms, seek support from others, and discuss concerns among the family unit.

1. Establish an open line of communication with the family, providing an atmosphere in which family members can ask questions, ventilate feelings, and discuss concerns among other family members.

2. Assess family members' knowledge about the patient's therapies and treatments. Provide information, as needed, and reinforce information the family has received from other health care members.

3. Provide opportunities and areas for family members to talk privately as well as share concerns with health care members.

4. Determine effective coping strategies that have been used by the family in other stressful situations. Support and encourage the family to continue use of healthy, effective coping strategies.

5. Enable family members to spend time alone with the patient for short, frequent intervals.

6. Encourage family members to pursue diversional activities outside the hospital to help alleviate stress of the immedi-

ate situation. Families often feel the need for "permission" from health care members to leave the waiting room or hospital.

7. Offer realistic hope.

# Chronic Respiratory Acidosis (Compensated)

Chronic respiratory acidosis is a disorder that occurs in pulmonary diseases (e.g., chronic emphysema and bronchitis) in which effective alveolar ventilation is decreased and a ventilation-perfusion mismatch is present. Chronic hypercapnia also can occur with obesity. In patients with a chronic lung disease, a nearly normal pH can be seen if renal function is normal, even if the $Paco_2$ is as high as 60 mm Hg. Chronic compensatory metabolic alkalosis (serum $HCO_3^-$ >28 mEq/L) occurs and maintains an acceptable acid-base environment, which results in compensated respiratory acidosis and a normal or near normal pH. Patients with chronic lung disease can experience acute rises in $Paco_2$ secondary to superimposed disease states such as pneumonia. If the chronic compensatory mechanisms in place (e.g., elevated $HCO_3^-$) are inadequate to meet the sudden increase in $Paco_2$, decompensation may occur with a resultant decrease in pH.

## Assessment

1. **Clinical manifestations:** If the $Paco_2$ does not exceed the body's ability to compensate, no specific findings will be noted. If $Paco_2$ rises rapidly, the following may occur: dull headache, weakness, dyspnea, asterixis, agitation, and insomnia progressing to somnolence and coma.

2. **Physical assessment:** Tachypnea and cyanosis. Severe hypercapnia ($Paco_2$ >70 mm Hg) may cause cerebral vasodilation resulting in increased ICP, papilledema, and dilated conjunctival and facial blood vessels. Depending on underlying pathophysiology, edema may be present secondary to right ventricular failure.

3. **History and risk factors:** See also the box on p. 161.
   - *Chronic obstructive pulmonary disease (COPD):* Predominantly emphysema and bronchitis.
   - *Extreme obesity:* Pickwickian syndrome.
   - *Development of superimposed acute respiratory infection in a patient with COPD.*

## Potential Causes of Chronic Respiratory Acidosis

**Obstructive Diseases**

Emphysema
Chronic bronchitis
Cystic fibrosis
Obstructive sleep apnea

**Restriction of Ventilation**

Kyphoscoliosis
Hydrothorax
Severe chronic pneu-
    monitis
Obesity-hypoventilation
    (Pickwickian) syndrome

**Neuromuscular Abnormalities**

Spinal cord injuries
Poliomyelitis
Muscular dystrophy
Multiple sclerosis
Amyotrophic lateral
    sclerosis (ALS)
Diaphragmatic paralysis
Myxedema

**Depression of the Respiratory Center**

Brain tumor
Bulbar poliomyelitis
Chronic sedative overdose

■ *Exposure to pulmonary toxins:* Occupational risk and pol-
lution.

## Diagnostic Tests

1. **ABG values:** Provide data necessary for determining the
diagnosis and severity of respiratory acidosis. Although the
$Paco_2$ will be elevated, the pH will be on the acidic (low) side
of normal because of renal compensation, except in patients
who are experiencing acute pulmonary infection. If the $Paco_2$
has increased abruptly from the baseline value, a pH lower
than normal may be seen.

2. **Total $CO_2$:** Serum $CO_2$ (equivalent to $HCO_3^-$) is especially
helpful in determining the level of metabolic compensation
that has occurred (i.e., increased $HCO_3^-$ with a near normal
pH if fully compensated). This information is particularly
useful in identifying "mixed" acid-base disturbances (see
Chapter 17) because the $HCO_3^-$ is expected to be elevated in
chronic respiratory acidosis. If the $HCO_3^-$ is normal or low,
this could be diagnostic of a pathologic process concurrent
with the respiratory acidosis.

3. **Chest x-ray:** Determines the extent of underlying pulmonary disease and identifies further pathologic changes that may be responsible for acute exacerbation (e.g., pneumonia).
4. **Electrocardiogram (ECG):** Identifies cardiac involvement from COPD. For example, right-sided heart failure is a complication of chronic bronchitis.
5. **Sputum culture:** Determines presence of pathogens causing an acute exacerbation of a chronic pulmonary disease (e.g., pneumonia) present in patients with COPD.

## Collaborative Management

1. **Oxygen therapy:** Used cautiously (i.e., not >3 L/min) in patients with chronic $CO_2$ retention for whom hypoxemia, rather than hypercapnia, stimulates ventilation. The patient may require intubation and mechanical ventilation for stupor and coma precipitated by oxygen if the drive to breathe is eliminated by high concentrations of oxygen.
2. **Pharmacotherapy:** Bronchodilators and antibiotics, as indicated. Narcotics and sedatives can depress the respiratory center and are avoided unless the patient is intubated and mechanically ventilated. Progesterone may be given as a respiratory stimulant; it is especially beneficial to obese patients.
3. **Intravenous (IV) fluids:** Maintain adequate hydration for mobilizing pulmonary secretions.
4. **Chest physiotherapy:** Aids in expectoration of sputum; includes postural drainage if hypersecretions are present. Assess the patient closely during this procedure because it may be poorly tolerated, especially the postural drainage component.

## Nursing Diagnoses and Interventions

**Impaired gas exchange** related to trapping of $CO_2$ secondary to pulmonary tissue destruction (appropriate for the patient with COPD).

**Desired outcome:** ABG values reflect a $Pa_{CO_2}$ and pH within an acceptable range, based on the patient's underlying pulmonary disease. Impairment of mental status or restlessness is absent or reduced.

1. Monitor serial ABG results to assess the patient's response

to therapy. Report significant findings to the physician: an increasing $Paco_2$ and a decreasing pH.

2. Assess and document the patient's respiratory status: RR and rhythm, exertional effort, and breath sounds. Compare pretreatment findings to posttreatment (e.g., oxygen therapy, physiotherapy, or medications) findings for evidence of improvement.

3. Assess and document the patient's LOC. If $Paco_2$ increases, be alert to subtle, progressive changes in mental status. A common progression is agitation→ insomnia→ somnolence→ coma. To avoid a comatose state secondary to rising $CO_2$ levels, always evaluate the arousability of a patient with elevated $Paco_2$ who appears to be sleeping. Notify the physician if the patient is difficult to arouse.

4. Ensure appropriate delivery of prescribed oxygen therapy. Assess the patient's respiratory status after every change in $Fio_2$. Patients with chronic $CO_2$ retention may be very sensitive to increases in $Fio_2$, resulting in depressed ventilatory drive. If the patient requires mechanical ventilation, be aware of the importance of maintaining the compensated acid-base environment. If the $Paco_2$ were rapidly decreased by a high RR per mechanical ventilation, a severe metabolic alkalosis could develop, resulting in severe neurologic abnormalities (e.g., seizures, coma). The sudden onset of metabolic alkalosis may also lead to hypocalcemia, which can result in tetany (see p. 109).

5. Assess for presence of bowel sounds and monitor for gastric distention, which can impede movement of the diaphragm and restrict ventilatory effort further.

6. If the patient is not intubated, encourage the use of pursed-lip breathing (inhalation through the nose, with slow exhalation through pursed lips), which helps airways remain open and allows for better air excursion. Optimally, this technique will diminish air entrapment in the lungs and make respiratory effort more efficient.

**Ineffective airway clearance** related to viscous secretions and fatigue.

**Desired outcome:** Auscultation of the patient's airway reveals the absence of adventitious breath sounds.

1. Be alert to increased fatigue or lethargy as a potential sign of increasing $Paco_2$.

2. If the patient is unable to raise secretions independently, perform suctioning as often as is determined by assessment findings.

3. If prescribed, administer chest physiotherapy. (Chest physiotherapy may be contraindicated in some patients with chronic $CO_2$ retention.) Evaluate the effectiveness of therapy by assessing breath sounds, ABG results, and patency of airway both before and after treatment.

4. Ensure adequate fluid intake to compensate for increased insensible losses caused by increased RR, febrile state, and diaphoresis. Adequate hydration will make secretions less viscous and easier to mobilize.

5. Encourage the nonintubated patient to continue with pursed-lip breathing (inhalation through the nose, with slow exhalation through pursed lips), which will increase efficiency and effectiveness of respiratory effort.

For other nursing diagnoses and interventions, see "Acute Respiratory Acidosis" for the following: "Altered oral mucous membrane related to abnormal breathing pattern" (see p. 158) and "Sleep pattern disturbance related to frequent treatments and procedures" (see pp. 158-159).

# Respiratory Alkalosis

## Acute Respiratory Alkalosis

Respiratory alkalosis occurs as a result of an increase in the rate of alveolar ventilation (alveolar hyperventilation). It is defined by a $Pa_{CO_2}$, partial pressure of carbon dioxide ($CO_2$) in arterial blood, less than 40 mm Hg (hypocapnia) and a pH greater than 7.40. Acute alveolar hyperventilation most frequently is the result of anxiety and is commonly referred to as hyperventilation syndrome. In addition, numerous physiologic disorders (see "History and risk factors," below) can cause acute hypocapnia, which results in increased pH. The rise in pH is modified to a small degree by intracellular buffering. To compensate for increased $CO_2$ loss and the resultant base excess, hydrogen ions are released from tissue buffers, which, in turn, lower plasma bicarbonate ($HCO_3^-$) concentration (a reduction of ~2 mEq/L/10 mm Hg decrease in partial pressure of carbon dioxide [$P_{CO_2}$]). The kidneys' response to respiratory alkalosis is slow (several hours to days), and thus acute respiratory alkalosis is usually resolved before renal compensation can occur.

## Assessment

1. **Clinical manifestations:** Lightheadedness, anxiety, paresthesias, and circumoral numbness. In extreme alkalosis, confusion, tetany, syncope, and seizures may occur.
2. **Physical assessment:** Increased rate and depth of respirations.
3. **Electrocardiogram (ECG) findings:** Cardiac dysrhythmias.
4. **History and risk factors** (see also the box on p. 166):
   - *Anxiety:* The patient is often unaware of hyperventilation.
   - *Acute hypoxemia:* Pulmonary disorders (e.g., pneumonia, mild to moderate asthmatic attack, pulmonary edema, and pulmonary thromboembolism) cause hypoxemia, which

## Potential Causes of Acute Respiratory Alkalosis

**Hypoxemia**
Pneumonia
High altitude (> 6500 feet)
Hypotension
Severe anemia
Congestive heart failure

**Pulmonary Disorders**
Pulmonary emboli
Inhalation of irritants
Interstitial fibrosis
Pulmonary edema
Asthma

**Central (Direct) Stimulation of the Respiratory Center**
Anxiety
Fever
Pain
Drugs (salicylates)
Voluntary or mechanical
  hyperventilation
Intracerebral trauma
Gram-negative septicemia
Acute cerebral vascular
  accident (unexplained
  respiratory alkalosis is a
  poor prognostic sign)

stimulates the ventilatory effort in the initial stages of the disease process.

- *Hypermetabolic states:* Fever and sepsis, especially gram-negative induced septicemia (respiratory alkalosis is an important early finding in septicemia).
- *Salicylate intoxication.*
- *Excessive mechanical ventilation.*
- *Central nervous system (CNS) trauma:* May result in damage to the respiratory center.

## Diagnostic Tests

1. **Arterial blood gas (ABG) values:** $Paco_2$ less than 40 mm Hg and pH greater than 7.40 will be present. A decreased oxygen tension of arterial blood ($Pao_2$), along with the clinical picture (e.g., pneumonia, pulmonary edema, pulmonary embolism, or adult respiratory distress syndrome), may help diagnose the etiology of the respiratory alkalosis. In patients spontaneously breathing, a $Paco_2$ less than 20 to 25 mm Hg may indicate a poor prognosis.

2. **Serum electrolytes:** Determine the presence of metabolic acid-base disorders. A $HCO_3^-$ concentration greater or less than a reduction of 2 mEq/L/10 mm Hg decrease in $Pco_2$

indicates a mixed acid-base imbalance (i.e., a metabolic alkalosis or acidosis).

3. **Serum phosphate:** May fall to less than 0.5 mg/dl (normal is 3 to 4.5 mg/dl) because of the alkalosis, which causes increased uptake of phosphate by the cells.

4. **ECG:** Detects cardiac dysrhythmias, which may be present with alkalosis.

## Collaborative Management

1. **Treatment of the underlying disorder.**

2. **Reassurance:** If anxiety is the cause of decreased $Paco_2$. If symptoms are severe, it may be necessary for the patient to rebreathe into a paper bag (this increases the $Pco_2$ in the inspired air). Instead of a paper bag, an oxygen mask with an attached $CO_2$ reservoir may be prescribed. It is important to recheck arterial pH to ensure metabolic acidosis does not occur from the decrease in $HCO_3^-$ as the $Pco_2$ returns to normal.

3. **Oxygen therapy:** If hypoxemia is the causative factor.

4. **Adjustments to mechanical ventilators:** Settings are checked and adjustments made to ventilatory parameters in response to ABG results that signal hypocapnia. Respiratory rate (RR) or volume is decreased and dead space is added, if necessary.

5. **Pharmacotherapy:** Sedatives and tranquilizers may be given for anxiety-induced respiratory alkalosis.

## Nursing Diagnoses and Interventions

**Ineffective breathing pattern** related to hyperventilation secondary to anxiety.

**Desired outcome:** The patient's breathing pattern is effective as evidenced by a $Paco_2$ of at least 35 mm Hg and a pH of 7.45 or lower.

1. To help alleviate anxiety, reassure the patient that a staff member will remain with him or her.

2. Encourage the patient to breathe slowly. Pace the patient's breathing by having him or her mimic your own breathing pattern.

3. Monitor the patient's cardiac rhythm, notifying the physician if dysrhythmias occur. With acute respiratory alkalosis, even a modest alkalosis can precipitate dysrhythmias in a patient

with a preexisting heart disease who is also taking cardiotropic drugs.

4. Administer sedatives or tranquilizers as prescribed.
5. Have the patient rebreathe into a paper bag or into an oxygen mask with an attached $CO_2$ reservoir, if prescribed.
6. Ensure that the patient rests undisturbed after his or her breathing pattern has stabilized. Hyperventilation can result in fatigue.

NOTE: Hyperventilation may lead to hypocalcemic tetany despite a normal or near normal calcium level because of increased binding of calcium (see Chapter 9).

# Chronic Respiratory Alkalosis

This is a state of chronic hypocapnia, which stimulates the renal compensatory response and results in a greater decrease in plasma $HCO_3^-$ (a reduction of 4 mEq/L/10 mm Hg decrease in $P_{CO_2}$). Maximal renal compensatory response requires several days to occur.

 Assessment

1. **Clinical manifestations:** Individuals with chronic respiratory alkalosis usually are asymptomatic.
2. **Physical assessment:** Increased RR and depth.
3. **History and risk factors:**
   - *Cerebral disease:* Tumor and encephalitis.
   - *Chronic hepatic insufficiency.*
   - *Pregnancy.*
   - *Chronic hypoxemia:* Adaptation to high altitude, cyanotic heart disease, and lung disease resulting in decreased compliance (e.g., fibrosis).

## Diagnostic Tests

1. **ABG values:** $Pa_{CO_2}$ will be less than 35 mm Hg, with a nearly normal pH; $Pa_{O_2}$ may be decreased if hypoxemia is the causative factor.
2. **Serum electrolytes:** Probably will be normal, with the exception of total $CO_2$ (serum $HCO_3^-$), which will decrease as renal compensation occurs. Maximal renal compensation takes 7 to 9 days with normalization of pH.

3. **Phosphate levels:** Hypophosphatemia (as low as 0.5 mg/dl) may be seen with intense hyperventilation. Alkalosis causes increased uptake of phosphate by the cells.

## Collaborative Management

1. **Treatment of the underlying cause.**
2. **Oxygen therapy:** If hypoxemia is present and identified as causative factor in respiratory alkalosis.

## Nursing Diagnoses and Interventions

Nursing diagnoses and interventions are specific to the pathophysiologic process.

# Metabolic Acidosis

# 15

## Acute Metabolic Acidosis

Metabolic acidosis is caused by a primary decrease in plasma bicarbonate, as reflected by a serum bicarbonate of less than 24 mEq/L with a pH less than 7.40. The decrease in serum bicarbonate is caused by one of the following mechanisms: (1) increase in the concentration of hydrogen ions in the form of nonvolatile acids (e.g., ketoacidosis associated with diabetes and alcoholism; lactic acidosis); (2) loss of alkali (e.g., severe diarrhea, intestinal malabsorption); or (3) decreased acid excretion by the kidneys (e.g., acute and chronic renal failure). The decrease in pH stimulates respirations. The body's attempts to compensate occur rapidly, as manifested by lowering of the partial pressure of carbon dioxide ($CO_2$) in arterial blood ($Paco_2$), which may be reduced by as much as 10 to 15 mm Hg. The most important mechanism for ridding the body of excess hydrogen ions ($H^+$) is the increase in acid excretion by the kidneys. However, nonvolatile acids may accumulate more rapidly than they can be neutralized by the body's buffers, compensated for by the respiratory system, or excreted by the kidneys. See Table 15-2 for a classification of acidosis.

### Assessment

1. **Clinical manifestations:** Findings vary, depending on underlying disease states and severity of acid-base disturbance. There may be changes in the level of consciousness that range from fatigue and confusion to stupor and coma.
2. **Physical assessment:** Decreased blood pressure, tachypnea leading to alveolar hyperventilation (Kussmaul's respirations), cold and clammy skin, presence of dysrhythmias, and shock state.
3. **History and risk factors** (see the box on p. 171):
   - *Renal disease*: Acute renal failure and renal tubular acidosis.

# Potential Causes of Metabolic Acidosis

**Loss of HCO$_3^-$**

Gastrointestinal
1. Diarrhea
2. Biliary and pancreatic drainage
3. Urethral sigmoidostomy or ileostomy
4. Cholestyramine

**Renal**

1. Renal tubular acidosis (RTA) type II
2. Carbonic anhydrase inhibitors (acetazalomide)

**Excess Acid Production/Ingestion**

Ketoacidosis
1. Diabetic
2. Alcohol induced

**Lactic Acidosis**

1. Hypercapnic metabolic acidosis

**Massive Rhabdomyolysis**

**Ingestion**

1. Salicylates*
2. Methanol (component of varnish, shellac)
3. Ethylene glycol (component of antifreeze)
4. Toluene (a component of paint thinner, model glue, and transmission fluid)
5. Hyperalimentation fluids if acetate or lactate is not added

**Inability of the Kidneys to Excrete Acid (H$^+$) Load**

**Renal Insufficiency; Acute or Chronic Renal Failure**

**RTA type I**

**Hypoaldosteronism**

**Potassium-Sparing Diuretics**

**Posthypercapneic Metabolic Acidosis (after correction of chronic respiratory alkalosis)**

*Pure metabolic acidosis is rare—usually a mixed acid base disorder.
$HCO_3^-$, Bicarbonate ion; $H^+$, hydrogen ion.

- *Ketoacidosis*: Diabetes mellitus, alcoholism, and starvation.
- *Lactic acidosis*: Respiratory or circulatory failure, drugs and toxins, hereditary disorders, and septic shock. It can be associated with other disease states such as leukemia, pancreatitis, bacterial infection, and uncontrolled diabetes mellitus.
- *Poisoning and drug toxicity*: Salicylates, methanol, ethylene glycol, and ammonium chloride.
- *Loss of alkali*: Draining wounds (e.g., pancreatic fistulas), diarrhea, ureterostomy, and cholestyramine.

## Diagnostic Tests

1. **Arterial blood gas (ABG) values:** Determine pH ($<7.40$) and degree of respiratory compensation as reflected by $Pa_{CO_2}$, which usually is less than 35 mm Hg. Increasing levels of $CO_2$ at the tissue level may not be reflected in ABGs even though overall $CO_2$ elimination is decreased (see #2).

2. **Mixed venous blood gases:** Help identify presence of hypercapnic metabolic acidosis. Mixed venous $CO_2$ will be markedly higher than arterial $P_{CO_2}$. The higher $CO_2$ is not related to impaired pulmonary function but is the result of the generation and accumulation of $CO_2$ at the cellular level during shock states, congestive heart failure, and cardiac arrest. Mixed venous gases should be obtained simultaneously with ABGs.

3. **Total $CO_2$:** Determines presence of metabolic acidosis (bicarbonate ion $[HCO_3^-]$ $<24$ mEq/L).

4. **Serum electrolytes:** Elevated potassium may be present because of the exchange of intracellular potassium for hydrogen ions in the body's attempt to normalize acid-base environment.

   - *Anion gap*: In attempting to identify the cause of metabolic acidosis, an analysis of serum electrolytes to detect anion gap may be helpful. Anion gap reflects unmeasureable anions present in plasma and is calculated by subtracting the sum of chloride and bicarbonate from the amount of plasma sodium concentration (Table 15-1). An increase in the anion gap is present with diabetic ketoacidosis,

Table 15-1    Anion gap

| Anion Gap Type | Values | Causes |
|---|---|---|
| Normal anion gap | 12 (±2) mEq/L | Diarrhea, renal tubular acidosis, or pancreatic fistula causing a direct loss of $HCO_3^-$; addition of chloride-containing acids |
| Increased anion gap | >14 mEq/L | Lactic acidosis, uremia, diabetic ketoacidosis (DKA), or salicylate and methanol toxicity, resulting in accumulation of nonvolatile acids with decrease in $HCO_3^-$ |

For more information about anion gap, see Chapter 5.

lactic acidosis, and other states when nonvolatile acids accumulate.

$$\text{Anion gap} = Na^+ - (Cl^- + HCO_3^-)$$

5. **Electrocardiogram (ECG):** Detects dysrhythmias caused by hyperkalemia. Changes seen with hyperkalemia include peaked T waves, depressed ST segment, decreased size of R waves, decrease or absence of P waves, and widened QRS complex. Acidosis can cause nonspecific ECG changes.

## Collaborative Management

1. **$NaHCO_3$:** May be indicated when arterial pH is 7.2 or lower. The usual mode of delivery is intravenous drip: 2 to 3 ampules (44.5 mEq/ampule) in 1000 ml 5% dextrose in water ($D_5W$). Concentration depends on severity of the acidosis and presence of any serum sodium disorders. $NaHCO_3$ must be given cautiously to avoid metabolic alkalosis and pulmonary edema secondary to the sodium

load. Use of $NaHCO_3^-$ is very controversial, especially when tissue hypoxia is present (i.e., shock, sepsis, cardiac arrest) because of the potential of worsening the acidosis (see #4 for treatment of the underlying disorder).

2. **Potassium replacement:** Usually, hyperkalemia is present, but a potassium deficit can occur as well. If a potassium deficit exists ($K^+$ <3.5), it must be corrected before $NaHCO_3$ is administered because when the acidosis is corrected, the potassium shifts back to intracellular spaces. This could result in serum hypokalemia with serious consequences such as cardiac irritability with fatal dysrhythmias and generalized muscle weakness (see Chapter 8 for more information).

3. **Mechanical ventilation:** If necessary, however, it is important that the patient's compensatory hyperventilation be allowed to continue to prevent acidosis from becoming more severe. Therefore the respiratory rate on the ventilator should not be set lower than the rate at which the patient has been breathing spontaneously, and the tidal volume should be large enough to maintain compensatory hyperventilation until the underlying disorder can be resolved.

4. **Treatment of the underlying disorder.**
   - *Diabetic ketoacidosis*: Insulin and fluids. If acidosis is severe (with a pH of <7.1 or $HCO_3^-$ 6 to 8 mEq/L), $NaHCO_3$ may be necessary, although its use is controversial.
   - *Alcoholism-related ketoacidosis*: Glucose and saline.
   - *Diarrhea*: Usually occurs in association with other fluid and electrolyte disturbances; correction addresses concurrent imbalances.
   - *Acute renal failure*: Hemodialysis or peritoneal dialysis to restore an adequate level of plasma bicarbonate (see Chapter 22).
   - *Renal tubular acidosis*: May require modest amounts (<100 mEq/day) of bicarbonate.
   - *Poisoning and drug toxicity*: Treatment depends on the drug ingested or infused. Hemodialysis or peritoneal dialysis may be necessary.
   - *Lactic acidosis*: Correction of the underlying disorder. Mortality associated with lactic acidosis is high. Use of $NaHCO_3$ is very controversial and may worsen acidosis if tissue hypoxia is present. $NaHCO_3$ may be given in small

amounts to keep pH higher than 7.10 with frequent monitoring of mixed venous pH.

## Nursing Diagnoses and Interventions

Nursing diagnoses and interventions are specific to the pathophysiologic process. In addition, see "Acute Respiratory Acidosis" for the following: "Sensory-perceptual alterations," p. 157; "Altered oral mucous membrane related to abnormal breathing pattern," p. 158; "Sleep pattern disturbance related to frequent treatments and procedures," p. 158; and "Ineffective family coping related to stress reaction," p. 159.

# Chronic Metabolic Acidosis

Most often, chronic metabolic acidosis is seen with chronic renal failure in which the kidneys' ability to excrete acids (endogenous and exogenous) is exceeded by acid production and ingestion. The $HCO_3^-$ in patients with end-stage renal failure usually decreases to 12 to 20 mEq/L. Treatment is indicated when serum bicarbonate levels reach 12 mEq/L. Respiratory compensation does occur, but to a limited degree. A modest decrease in $Paco_2$ will be noted on ABG values. See Table 15-2 for a classification of acidosis.

## Assessment

1. **Clinical manifestations:** Usually the patient is asymptomatic, although fatigue, malaise, and anorexia may be present in relation to the underlying disease.
2. **History and risk factors:** Chronic renal failure and renal tubular acidosis.

## Diagnostic Tests

1. **ABG values:** $Paco_2$ will be less than 35 mm Hg; pH will be less than 7.40 (in advanced renal failure, the pH is ≈7.30 or higher).
2. **Total $CO_2$:** Will be less than 24 mEq/L (usually 12 to 18 mEq/L). With severe acidosis, it will be 12 mEq/L or lower.
3. **Serum electrolytes:** The serum calcium level is checked before treatment of acidosis is initiated to prevent tetany induced by hypocalcemia (caused by a decrease in ionized calcium). The serum potassium level should be monitored

**Table 15-2**  Classification of acidosis

| | Control | Classification of Acidosis | | | |
|---|---|---|---|---|---|
| | | Metabolic Acidosis with Normal Anion Gap | Metabolic Acidosis with Elevated Anion Gap | Hypercapnic Metabolic Acidosis | |
| Arterial pH | 7.35-7.45 | Below 7.35 | Below 7.35 | Below 7.35 | |
| Arterial $P_{CO_2}$ | 35-45 mm Hg | Low | Low | Normal to high | |
| Mixed venous $P_{CO_2}$ | 41-51 mm Hg | Low | Low | Much higher than arterial $P_{CO_2}$ | |
| Blood bicarbonate | 22-26 mmol/L | Low | Low | Low | |
| Blood chloride | 95-108 mmol/L | Elevated | Normal | Normal | |
| Anion gap (Na) − (Cl + bicarbonate) | 10-14 mmol/L | Normal to low | Elevated | Elevated | |
| Major source of excess [$H^+$] ion | — | Normal metabolism | Endogenous or exogenous non-volatile acids | Hydrolysis of adenosine triphosphate, carbonic acid, lactic acid | |
| Clinical examples | — | Renal tubular acidosis | Uremia, diabetic ketoacidosis | Cardiac arrest, congestive heart failure | |

Modified from Parrillo J, Bone R: *Critical care medicine: principles of diagnosis and management*, St Louis, 1995, Mosby.

after acidosis has been corrected to detect hypokalemia because potassium shifts back into the cells.

## Collaborative Management

1. **Alkalizing agents:** For serum bicarbonate levels less than 12 mEq/L, oral alkali are administered ($NaHCO_3$ tablets). They are used cautiously to prevent fluid overload and tetany caused by hypocalcemia. Sodium citrate should be avoided because it may increase aluminum absorption. (This is a particular problem if aluminum hydroxide is used to control hyperphosphatemia.) NOTE: Be alert to the possibility of pulmonary edema if oliguria is present and bicarbonate is administered parenterally. Chronic acidosis is of concern in chronic renal failure because the bones are used as a chronic buffer and this contributes to renal bone disease. Metabolic acidosis can also lead to increased skeletal muscle break-down, leading to weakness. Metabolic acidoses causes an increase in ammonium production, which can lead to nephron injury, which speeds up progression of kidney disease.

2. **Hemodialysis or peritoneal dialysis:** If indicated by chronic renal failure or other disease processes. Uncontrolled acidosis may be an indicator of the need for initiating or increasing dialytic therapy in the patient with chronic renal failure.

## Nursing Diagnoses and Interventions

*ndx:*

**Altered nutrition:** Less than body requirements related to decreased intake secondary to fatigue, dietary restrictions, and metallic taste in the mouth (caused by uremic state).

**Desired outcome:** The patient's weight remains stable.

1. Provide foods that correspond to the patient's prescribed diet and preference.
2. Offer small meals and snacks at frequent intervals.
3. Offer oral care often to minimize the metallic taste. Brushing teeth before meals and using mouthwash frequently throughout the day are helpful.
4. Provide hard candy to keep the oral mucosa moist, diminish metallic taste, and supply calories.
5. Monitor hemoglobin and hematocrit levels to determine if anemia may be contributing to the patient's fatigue.

6. Provide periods of uninterrupted rest by clustering necessary treatments and procedures. If possible, avoid performing unpleasant or uncomfortable treatments 1 hour before and after mealtimes.

7. Encourage family members to eat with the patient or be present at mealtimes to provide social interaction.

Other nursing diagnoses and interventions are specific to the underlying pathophysiologic process.

# Metabolic Alkalosis

# 16

## Acute Metabolic Alkalosis

Acute metabolic alkalosis is a disorder that results in an elevated serum bicarbonate greater than 24 mEq/L and a pH greater than 7.40 as a result of hydrogen ion loss or excess alkali intake. A compensatory increase in partial pressure of carbon dioxide in arterial blood ($Paco_2$) (up to 50 to 60 mm Hg) will be seen. Respiratory compensation is limited because of hypoxemia, which develops secondary to decreased alveolar ventilation. The major causes of acute metabolic alkalosis are loss of gastric acid from vomiting or nasogastric (NG) suction and diuretic use. Posthypercapneic alkalosis (which occurs when chronic carbon dioxide [$CO_2$] retention is corrected rapidly) and excessive sodium bicarbonate administration (i.e., overcorrection of a metabolic acidosis) are less common causes.

## Assessment

1. **Clinical manifestations:** Muscular weakness, neuromuscular instability, hyporeflexia, polyuria, and polydipsia occur secondary to accompanying hypokalemia. Signs of volume depletion (i.e., postural hypotension, decreased jugular venous pressure, poor skin turgor) may also be present. Severe alkalosis can result in signs of neuromuscular excitability as well as apathy, confusion, and stupor.
2. **Electrocardiogram (ECG) findings:** Numerous types of atrial-ventricular dysrhythmias as a result of the cardiac irritability occurring with hypokalemia; changes in the T and U waves.
3. **History and risk factors:** See the box on p. 180.
   - *Clinical circumstances associated with volume/chloride depletion:* Vomiting or gastric drainage.
   - *Posthypercapneic alkalosis.*

## Potential Causes of Metabolic Alkalosis

### $H^+$ Loss

1. Gastrointestinal
   - Loss of gastric secretions (NG suctioning or vomiting)*
   - Villous adenoma
   - Congenital chloridorrhea
2. Renal
   - Diuretics (especially *loop* and thiazides*)
   - Mineralocorticoid excess*
   - Postchronic hypercapnia
   - Carbenicillin/penicillin derivation
   - Hypercalcemia/hypoparathyroidism
3. $H^+$ shift into the cells
   - Hypokalemia*
   - Carbohydrate refeeding after starvation

### $HCO_3^-$ Retention

1. Administration of large doses of bicarbonate or bicarbonate precursors
2. Massive blood transfusion
3. Milk-alkali syndrome

### Contraction Alkalosis

Diuretics
Cystic fibrosis

*Most common causes.
$H^+$, Hydrogen; *NG*, nasogastric; $HCO_3^-$, bicarbonate ion.

- *Excessive alkali intake:* May be iatrogenic from overcorrection of metabolic acidosis (frequently seen during cardiopulmonary resuscitation [CPR]). Excessive ingestion of sodium bicarbonate (e.g., Alka-Seltzer) or calcium carbonate (e.g., Tums, Rolaids) is another potential cause if renal insufficiency is already present and bicarbonate ion ($HCO_3^-$) excretion is affected.
- *Acute, aggressive thiazide diuretic therapy.*
- *Surreptitious vomiting or diuretic use:* If no cause is apparent, this must be considered.

# Diagnostic Tests

1. **Arterial blood gas (ABG) values:** Determine severity of alkalosis and response to therapy. The pH will be greater than 7.40. In severe metabolic alkalosis, the $Paco_2$ can exceed 60 mm Hg, as a compensatory response (in the absence of underlying lung disease).

2. **Total $CO_2$:** Values will be elevated to greater than 28 mEq/L.

3. **Serum electrolytes:** Usually, serum potassium ($K^+$) will be low (<4 mEq/L) as will serum chloride ($Cl^-$) (<95 mEq/L). Although the relationship between metabolic alkalosis and $K^+$ is not completely understood, alkalosis and hypokalemia often occur together.

4. **Urine $Cl^-$:** Helps differentiate between causes of metabolic alkalosis.

5. **ECG:** To assess for dysrhythmias, especially if profound alkalosis or hypokalemia is present.

# Collaborative Management

Management depends on the underlying disorder. Mild or moderate metabolic alkalosis usually does not require specific therapeutic interventions.

1. **Saline infusion:** Normal saline infusion may correct volume ($Cl^-$) deficit in patients with alkalosis secondary to gastric losses. Metabolic alkalosis is difficult to correct if hypovolemia and $Cl^-$ deficit are not corrected.

2. **Potassium chloride (KCl):** Indicated for patients with low $K^+$ levels. KCl is preferred over other $K^+$ salts because $Cl^-$ losses can be replaced simultaneously.

3. **Sodium and KCl:** Effective for posthypercapneic alkalosis, which occurs when chronic $CO_2$ retention is corrected rapidly (e.g., via mechanical ventilation). If adequate amounts of $Cl^-$ and $K^+$ are not available, renal excretion of excess bicarbonate is impaired and metabolic alkalosis continues.

4. **Histamine $H_2$ receptor antagonists (e.g., cimetidine, ranitidine, and famotidine):** Reduce production of gastric hydrochloric acid (HCl) and therefore are useful in preventing or decreasing the metabolic alkalosis that can occur with gastric suctioning.

5. **Carbonic anhydrase inhibitors:** Acetazolamide (Diamox) is especially useful for correcting metabolic alkalosis for

patients who cannot tolerate rapid volume expansion (e.g., individuals with congestive heart failure). It can be given orally or intravenously. Acetazolamide causes a large increase in renal secretion of $HCO_3^-$ and $K^+$, and therefore it may be necessary to supplement potassium before giving the drug.

6. **Acidifying agents:** Severe metabolic alkalosis (pH of >7.60 and $HCO_3^-$ 40 to 45 mEq/L) may require treatment with acidifying agents such as diluted HCl, ammonium chloride, or arginine hydrochloride. Because of their serious side effects, these medications are rarely used.

## *ndx:* Nursing Diagnoses and Interventions

Nursing diagnoses and interventions are specific to the underlying pathophysiologic process. In addition, the following may apply.
**Decreased cardiac output** related to electric factors (risk of dysrhythmias) secondary to metabolic alkalosis induced by gastric suctioning or potassium-wasting diuretics.
**Desired outcome:** ECG reveals a normal tracing; pH is 7.45 or lower.

1. Monitor laboratory values, especially pH and serum $CO_2$ to determine the patient's response to therapy. Notify the physician if there are significant changes or a lack of response to treatment.

2. Monitor ECG for the presence of dysrhythmias. Assess apical and radial pulses simultaneously when evaluating cardiac rate and rhythm to detect pulse deficit. Notify the physician of any changes in cardiac rate and rhythm.

3. Monitor $K^+$ levels, especially in patients receiving digitalis preparations. (Recall that hypokalemia frequently coexists with metabolic alkalosis.) Notify the physician if $K^+$ levels drop below 3.5 mEq/L. Hypokalemia sensitizes patients to the cardiotoxic effect of digitalis.

4. Use isotonic saline solutions to irrigate gastric tubes. Water is not recommended for irrigation because it can cause a washout of electrolytes.

5. If the patient is permitted to have ice chips, administer limited quantities to avoid washing electrolytes from the patient's stomach. Total volume of ice consumed over a shift frequently is underestimated. Determine the volume of a specific number of ice cubes or the quantity of crushed ice

by melting and measuring. Establish the volume of fluid the patient may consume each shift. Document the volume consumed in milliliters or ounces not by the number of cubes.

6. Measure and document the amount of fluid removed by suction.

7. Weigh the patient daily to determine fluid volume status.

8. Administer histamine $H_2$ receptor antagonist (e.g., cimetadine, ranitidine, or famotidine) as prescribed to block hydrochloride secretion by the stomach, thus lessening systemic metabolic alkalosis.

9. Monitor and record the patient's rate and depth of respirations. Diuretic-induced metabolic alkalosis eliminates the force acidemia normally would exert to sustain the respiratory drive, resulting in the potential for compromised respirations. NOTE: This disorder usually is not seen in the alert patient.

## Chronic Metabolic Alkalosis

Chronic metabolic alkalosis results in a pH greater than 7.40. $Paco_2$ will be elevated (>45 mm Hg) to compensate for the loss of hydrogen ion ($H^+$) or excess serum $HCO_3^-$. There are three clinical situations in which this can occur: (1) abnormalities in the kidneys' excretion of $HCO_3^-$ related to a mineralcorticoid effect, (2) loss of $H^+$ through the gastrointestinal (GI) tract, and (3) diuretic therapy.

### Assessment

1. **Clinical manifestations:** The patient may be asymptomatic. With severe $K^+$ depletion and profound alkalosis, the patient may experience weakness, neuromuscular instability, and decrease in GI tract motility, which can result in ileus.

2. **ECG findings:** Frequent premature ventricular contractions or U waves with hypokalemia and alkalosis.

3. **History and risk factors**
   - *Diuretic use:* Thiazide diuretics cause a loss of $Cl^-$, $K^+$, and $H^+$. Massive depletion of $K^+$ stores with loss of up to 1000 mEq, which is one third of total body $K^+$, may occur causing profound hypokalemia ($K^+ \leq 2$ mEq).
   - *Hyperadrenocorticism:* Cushing's syndrome and primary aldosteronism will cause a mild to moderate alkalosis. More severe alkalosis will be seen with adrenocortico-

tropic hormone secreting tumors (bronchogenic carcinoma). Not a $Cl^-$ deficit but a chronic loss of $K^+$, which can lead to total body depletion of $K^+$ with profound hypokalemia ($K^+ \leq 2$ mEq/L).

- *Chronic vomiting or chronic GI losses through gastric suction.*
- *Milk alkali syndrome:* An infrequent cause of metabolic alkalosis. Hypercalcemic nephropathy and alkalosis develop secondary to excessive intake of absorbable alkali.
- *Cystic fibrosis:* Large amounts of $Cl^-$ can be lost through sweat.

## Diagnostic Tests

1. **ABG values:** Determine severity of acid-base imbalance. $Paco_2$ will be increased (>45 mm Hg) and pH will be greater than 7.40.
2. **Total $CO_2$:** Will be greater than 28 mEq/L.
3. **Serum electrolytes:** Usually, $K^+$ will be profoundly low (may be $\leq 2$ mEq/L). $Cl^-$ may be less than 95 mEq/L and magnesium may be less than 1.5 mEq/L. Hypomagnesemia may contribute to irritability of the myocardium.

## Collaborative Management

The goal is to correct the underlying acid-base disorder via the following interventions.

1. **Fluid management:** If volume depletion exists, normal saline infusions are given.
2. **Potassium replacement:** If a $Cl^-$ deficit is also present, KCl is the drug of choice. If a $Cl^-$ deficit does not exist, other $K^+$ salts are acceptable.
   - *Intravenous potassium:* If the patient is on a cardiac monitor, up to 20 mEq/hr of KCl is given for serious hypokalemia. Concentrated doses of KCl (>40 mEq/L) require administration through a central venous line because of blood vessel irritation.
   - *Oral potassium:* Tastes *very* unpleasant. Most patients can tolerate only 15 mEq per glass, with a maximum daily dose of 60 to 80 mEq. Slow-release potassium tablets are an acceptable form of KCl. All forms of KCl may be irritating to gastric or intestinal mucosa.

- *Dietary:* Normal diet contains 3 g or 75 mEq of $K^+$ but not in the form of KCl. Dietary supplementation of $K^+$ is not effective if a concurrent $Cl^-$ deficit is also present.
3. **Potassium-sparing diuretics:** May be added to treatment if thiazide diuretics are the cause of hypokalemia and metabolic alkalosis.
4. **Identify and correct the cause of hyperadrenocorticism.**

## Nursing Diagnoses and Interventions

*ndx:*

**Knowledge deficit:** Necessary precautions for taking thiazide diuretics.

**Desired outcome:** The patient verbalizes knowledge about thiazide diuretics and the necessary precautions that must be taken.

1. Provide the patient and significant others with the following information about the prescribed thiazide diuretic: name, purpose, dosage, precautions, and potential side effects.
2. Stress the importance of taking only the prescribed dose because higher concentrations of the medication increase the risk of hypokalemia and alkalosis.
3. Explain that diets high in sodium increase the risk of alkalosis and hypokalemia, necessitating restrictions of sodium as prescribed.
4. If KCl supplements are prescribed, teach the patient the following:
   - Oral potassium has an unpleasant taste and is most palatable when mixed with orange juice or tomato juice.
   - Slow-release tablets should not be chewed.
   - Oral potassium and slow-release potassium tablets can irritate the stomach and should be taken with meals.
   - Although many foods contain potassium, they should not be used as a substitute for the KCl supplements prescribed by the patient's physician.

For other nursing diagnoses and interventions, see "Acute Metabolic Alkalosis" for the following: "Decreased cardiac output related to electric factors (risk of dysrhythmias) secondary to metabolic alkalosis induced by gastric suctioning or potassium-wasting diuretics," p. 182.

# Mixed Acid-Base Disorders

**17**

## Mixed Acid-Base Disorders

A mixed acid-base disturbance occurs when two or more simple acid-base disorders are present at the same time. The effect of a mixed acid-base disturbance on the pH depends on both the specific disorders involved and their severity. If a mixed disorder involves two types of acidosis, a larger drop in pH can be expected than would occur if a mixed acidosis-alkalosis disorder were present. When two opposing disorders (i.e., an acidosis and an alkalosis) occur simultaneously, the pH will be determined by the predominant disorder. In some cases the pH will be normal in the presence of a mixed acid-base disorder (Table 17-1).

### Case Study One

The patient has a history of chronic obstructive pulmonary disease (COPD) with carbon dioxide retention and is admitted after 3 days of diarrhea. The patient's normal response to an increased partial pressure of carbon dioxide in arterial blood ($Pa_{CO_2}$) (respiratory acidosis) is a compensatory increase in serum bicarbonate ion ($HCO_3^-$).

### Values

| pH | $Pa_{CO_2}$ | $HCO_3^-$ |
|----|-------------|-----------|
| 7.23 | 65 mm Hg | 29 mEq/L |

### Evaluation

The loss of bicarbonate secondary to the diarrhea leads to a decreased $HCO_3^-$ with a concomitant metabolic acidosis. Although

Table 17-1   Mixed acid-base disorders

| Types | Examples |
|---|---|
| Metabolic acidosis and metabolic acidosis | Renal failure, diarrhea |
| Acute respiratory acidosis and chronic respiratory acidosis | Pneumonia, emphysema |
| Metabolic acidosis and metabolic alkalosis | Diabetic ketoacidosis, vomiting |
| Metabolic acidosis and respiratory acidosis | Lactic acidosis, respiratory arrest |
| Metabolic acidosis and respiratory alkalosis | Ethylene glycol ingestion, pneumonia |
| Metabolic alkalosis and respiratory acidosis | Gastric suction, sedative overdose |
| Metabolic alkalosis and respiratory alkalosis | Diuretic use, hepatic failure |

the $HCO_3^-$ remains higher than normal, it is lower than would be expected for this patient. These values, with the patient's history, reflect a mixed acid-base disorder: respiratory acidosis and metabolic acidosis.

## Case Study Two

The patient is admitted with a history of cirrhosis and prolonged diarrhea.

## Values

| pH | $Pa_{CO_2}$ | $Na^+$ | $K^+$ | $Cl^-$ | $HCO_3^-$ | Anion gap |
|---|---|---|---|---|---|---|
| 7.38 | 28 | 138 | 2.9 | 115 | 13 | 10 |

$Na^+$   $Cl^-$   $HCO_3^-$
Anion gap determination: $138 - (115 + 13) = 10$

## Evaluation

Cirrhosis stimulates the respiratory center, resulting in respiratory alkalosis. Prolonged diarrhea has resulted in the loss of $HCO_3^-$, leading to metabolic acidosis with a normal anion gap. Over time, respiratory alkalosis can result in a compensatory decrease in serum $HCO_3^-$, but normally serum $HCO_3^-$ does not decrease to less than 16 mEq/L as a compensatory measure. Therefore these values, along with the patient's history, reflect a mixed acid-base disorder: respiratory alkalosis and metabolic acidosis. The pH is in the normal range because the opposing disorders, respiratory alkalosis and metabolic acidosis, have "balanced" each other.

## Case Study Three

The patient is an 80-year-old male who is 3 days posttransurethral resection, with nausea, slight confusion, and a temperature of 38.9°C (102°F).

## Values

| pH | $Pa_{CO_2}$ | $Na^+$ | $K^+$ | $Cl^-$ | $HCO_3^-$ | Anion gap |
|----|-------------|--------|-------|--------|-----------|-----------|
| 7.41 | 30 | 140 | 3.7 | 95 | 19 | 26 |

$Na^+$   $Cl^-$   $HCO_3^-$
Anion gap determination: $140 - (95 + 19) = 26$

## Evaluation

Sepsis-induced stimulation of the respiratory center leads to respiratory alkalosis. Metabolic acidosis results from lactic acid production and accumulation caused by tissue hypoxia from vaso-dilation secondary to septic shock. The presence of an increased anion gap (>14) signals the addition of nonvolatile acids to the system, indicating that the decreased $HCO_3^-$ is not a renal compensatory response to the respiratory alkalosis. These values, along with the patient's history, reflect a mixed acid-base disorder: respiratory alkalosis and anion gap metabolic acidosis. NOTE: Respiratory alkalosis is often an early, subtle sign of the onset of serious illness or complication in a hospitalized patient.

## Case Study Four

Twenty minutes ago the patient experienced a cardiac arrest secondary to ventricular dysrhythmias. The patient was given 2 ampules of sodium bicarbonate and is being ventilated manually at a rate of 24 breaths/min.

## Values

| pH | Paco$_2$ | HCO$_3^-$ |
|----|----------|-----------|
| 7.65 | 28 | 36 |

## Evaluation

The elevated serum HCO$_3^-$ is a result of overadministration of sodium bicarbonate during resuscitation and is the cause of the metabolic alkalosis. The respiratory alkalosis that *is* present has occurred because of the manual hyperventilation. Based on the patient's history and laboratory values, the patient has a mixed acid-base disorder: metabolic alkalosis and respiratory alkalosis.

Routine administration of sodium bicarbonate is no longer recommended for cardiac arrest.

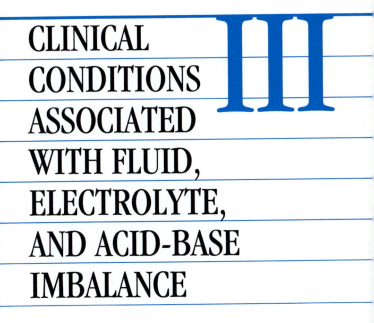

# CLINICAL CONDITIONS ASSOCIATED WITH FLUID, ELECTROLYTE, AND ACID-BASE IMBALANCE

**III**

# Gastrointestinal Disorders

18

As stated in Chapter 3, the gastrointestinal (GI) tract plays an important role in maintaining fluid and electrolyte balance because, in health, it is the primary site of fluid and electrolyte gain. Approximately 1.5 to 2 L of fluid are gained each day through the consumption of fluids and solid food. In addition, approximately 6 L of fluid are secreted into and reabsorbed out of the GI tract daily, equaling approximately half of the extracellular fluid (ECF) volume. Despite this large volume, the GI tract contributes minimally to normal fluid loss (approximately 100 to 200 ml/day). In disease, however, the GI tract becomes the most common site of abnormal fluid and electrolyte loss, potentially resulting in profound fluid and electrolyte imbalance.

The composition of the GI secretions varies with the location within the GI tract (Table 18-1). Therefore the nature of the fluid and electrolyte imbalance will vary with the type of fluid lost. GI fluids include saliva and bile, as well as gastric, pancreatic, and intestinal secretions. GI disorders causing fluid and electrolyte loss may be differentiated into loss of upper GI contents and loss of lower GI contents.

## Loss of Upper Gastrointestinal Contents

Upper GI secretions include saliva and gastric juices. Losses may occur because of problems such as vomiting and procedures such as gastric suction. See the box on p. 195 for potential causes of vomiting.

### Saliva

Approximately 1 L of saliva is produced each day. Saliva begins the digestive process by initiating the breakdown of starches. In addition, it lubricates food, facilitating swallowing. Food and saliva move through the esophagus to the stomach by means of peristalsis

Table 18-1   Volume and composition of gastrointestinal secrections*

| Secretion | Liter/24° | $Na^+$ (mEq/L) | $K^+$ (mEq/L) | $Cl^-$ (mEq/L) | $HCO_3^-$ (mEq/L) |
|---|---|---|---|---|---|
| Saliva | 1 | 40 | 15 | 30 | 0 |
| Gastric juice | 1-2 | 40 | 7 | 100 | 0 |
| Pancreatic juice | 1-2 | 130 | 7 | 60 | 100 |
| Bile | 1 | 150 | 7 | 80 | 30 |
| Intestinal secretions | 1-2 | 140 | 5 | Variable | Variable |

*Values are approximate.

## Potential Causes of Vomiting

- Gastrointestinal infection
- Inner ear infection
- Certain medications (e.g., chemotherapy)
- Pregnancy
- Small bowel obstruction
- Pyloric stenosis
- Uremia
- Binge-purge syndrome
- Pancreatitis
- Hepatitis
- Diabetic ketoacidosis

(rhythmic contractions). Once in the stomach, the food and saliva are exposed to the acidic secretions found there (see "Gastric Juices," below). Abnormal loss of saliva may occur in individuals who are unable to swallow their oral secretions (e.g., those who are comatose).

## Gastric Juices

Approximately 1 to 2 L of gastric juices are produced daily and contain hydrochloric acid, which aids digestion by breaking down food; the enzyme pepsin, which initiates digestion of proteins; and intrinsic factor, which facilitates the absorption of vitamin $B_{12}$ in the ileum.

Only alcohol and a limited amount of water are absorbed from the stomach. Most of the stomach contents move by peristalsis into the small intestine. Although the fluid and electrolyte content of food is variable, gastric contents mix and become similar in concentration to the ECF because of osmotic shifts of water into and out of the stomach. Losses from the upper GI tract (above the pylorus) are essentially isotonic and contain sodium, potassium, chloride, and hydrogen (see Table 18-1).

## Gastric Suction

Gastric suction, whether via a nasogastric or orogastric tube, is a common medical procedure used to decompress the stomach. Removal of gastric contents may lead to multiple fluid and electrolyte imbalances and requires adequate parenteral replacement. This may be accomplished by administering an intravenous solution developed specifically for gastric replacement (e.g., Isolyte G made by McGaw) or customizing a solution to meet the individual patient's needs, based on serum electrolyte levels. The following are nursing considerations that are important for minimizing electrolyte imbalance with gastric suction:

- **Give the patient nothing by mouth.**
- **Avoid giving ice by mouth or irrigating the catheter with plain water** because these actions will increase the loss of electrolytes because of "wash out." If patients are allowed ice chips, give small amounts (<1 oz) hourly.
- **Provide frequent oral care** to minimize thirst and maximize comfort.
- **Irrigate the gastric tube with isotonic sodium chloride (NaCl) solution only.** If the catheter is irrigated and an equal amount is not withdrawn and discarded, the extra irrigant should be added to the intake record to avoid overestimation of the fluid loss.

## Potential Fluid, Electrolyte, and Acid-Base Disturbances with Loss of Upper Gastrointestinal Contents

1. **Hypovolemia** caused by abnormal fluid loss (see Chapter 6).
2. **Hyponatremia** caused by loss of sodium-rich fluids with inadequate electrolyte replacement; and/or caused by antidiuretic hormone (ADH) and thirst-induced retention of water (see Chapter 7).
3. **Hypokalemia** caused by loss of potassium-containing fluids with inadequate replacement. Increased production of aldosterone secondary to hypovolemia will contribute to the development of hypokalemia caused by increased renal losses. Remember that aldosterone causes both an increased retention of sodium and increased excretion of potassium (see Chapter 8).
4. **Hypomagnesemia** as the result of prolonged loss of upper GI fluids with inadequate replacement (see Chapter 11).
5. **Metabolic alkalosis** caused by the loss of fluids rich in chloride and hydrogen. Hypovolemia contributes to the development and perpetuation of metabolic alkalosis as a result of volume-induced conservation of sodium bicarbonate ($NaHCO_3$) (see Chapter 16).

# Loss of Lower Gastrointestinal Contents

The small intestines are the primary site of nutrient, electrolyte, and water absorption. Approximately 6 L of fluid enter the small intestines from the upper GI tract daily, of which 75% is absorbed (and returned to the ECF). The colon receives only 1 to 2 L of fluid from the ileum; of this, normally all are absorbed except 100 to 200 ml of water and a small quantity of electrolytes.

Losses from the lower GI tract (below the pylorus) are generally isotonic and contain sodium, potassium, and bicarbonate. Lower GI contents may be lost through diarrhea, intestinal fistulas, or intestinal resection. Abnormal losses from the small intestines of as much as 2000 ml/day may occur with the creation of a new ileostomy or with short bowel syndrome. Although the loss of water and electrolytes remains greater than that with normal stool, over time, ileostomy output decreases to only 300 to 500 ml/day. Fistulas (an abnormal passage from the bowel to the skin) also may result in the loss of several liters of intestinal fluid daily. Diarrhea, however, remains the most common cause of lower GI fluid loss, especially in children. In developed countries, diarrhea accounts for a significant percentage of pediatric hospital admissions and clinic visits. In underdeveloped nations, diarrhea is a major cause of infant deaths (see "Diarrhea," p. 198, and the box below).

Vomiting can contribute to lower GI fluid loss because both gastric and duodenal contents may be lost. Losses from both the

## Potential Causes of Diarrhea

**Osmotic Diarrhea**
- Certain medications (e.g., lactulose, sorbitol)
- Malabsorption or maldigestion syndromes

**Secretory Diarrhea**
- Gastrointestinal infection
- Inflammatory bowel disease
- Emotional stress
- Pancreatic insufficiency
- Intestinal obstruction
- Abuse of laxatives (e.g., bisacodyl, castor oil)
- Carcinoma

upper and lower GI tract also can occur with bowel obstruction. Acid-base balance usually is maintained when both gastric and duodenal fluids are lost because a loss of both hydrogen (acid) and bicarbonate (base) occurs.

Lower GI secretions include bile, pancreatic juice, and intestinal secretions (succus entericus).

## Pancreatic Juice

Approximately 1 to 2 L of pancreatic juice are secreted each day. Pancreatic juice is high in bicarbonate, which neutralizes the acidic gastric contents as they enter the duodenum. It also contains enzymes that aid in the digestion of protein (trypsin), starches (amylase), and fats (lipase).

## Bile

Bile is produced by the liver and stored in the gallbladder. Water and electrolytes are continuously reabsorbed by the gallbladder mucosa so that the bile released into the duodenum may be five to ten times more concentrated than the bile produced by the liver. The liver produces approximately 1 L of bile per day. Bile provides a means of excreting bilirubin (a breakdown product of hemoglobin) and aids in the digestion of fats via emulsification by bile salts. In addition to bilirubin and bile salts, bile contains water, sodium, potassium, calcium, bicarbonate, cholesterol, and lecithin.

## Intestinal Secretions

In addition to bile and pancreatic juice, the intestines contain secretions produced by the intestinal glands. These glands secrete mucus, which helps protect the intestinal mucosa, hormones (e.g., secretin), electrolytes, and digestive enzymes. Approximately 1 to 2 L of intestinal gland secretions are produced each day. The secretion of isotonic intestinal fluids may increase dramatically in certain diseases such as cholera and other intestinal infections, after administration of certain medications such as laxatives, and with bowel obstruction (see "Bowel Obstruction," on p. 199).

## Diarrhea

*Diarrhea* is defined as an increased loss of fluid and electrolytes via the stool. The causes of diarrhea are divided into two main categories: (1) those causing osmotic diarrhea and (2) those causing secretory diarrhea. Osmotic diarrhea occurs when poorly absorbable solutes are present in the colon. The unabsorbed solutes create an osmotic gradient for water to move from the ECF into the lumen of the bowel. In addition, water that normally would be reabsorbed from the bowel remains in the lumen. This is the means by which sorbitol and lactulose induce diarrhea. Malabsorption or maldigestion of carbohydrates also will result in osmotic diarrhea because bacteria in the colon convert unabsorbed carbohydrates to organic acids. These organic acids create an osmotic gradient favoring the production of liquid stools. Osmotic diarrhea usually stops within 24 to 48 hours of fasting.

Water and electrolytes are both secreted into and reabsorbed from the lumen of the bowel. Under normal conditions there is net reabsorption, minimizing the volume of the stool. Secretory diarrhea develops when there is either increased secretion or decreased reabsorption of water and electrolytes. Unlike osmotic diarrhea, secretory diarrhea does not cease with fasting and is characterized by large losses of water and electrolytes. Bacterial infections cause secretory diarrhea by irritating the bowel mucosa and causing increased secretion of water and electrolytes. The diarrhea that occurs with inflammatory bowel diseases (ulcerative colitis and Crohn's disease) is believed to be the result of inflammation of the bowel wall, which causes both an increase in the secretion and decrease in reabsorption. The individual with inflammatory bowel disease may pass more than five stools a day, causing both physical and emotional debilitation.

## Bowel Obstruction

The type and extent of fluid and electrolyte imbalance that occurs with bowel obstruction depends on the location of the obstruction and its duration. The longer the bowel is obstructed, the more profound the fluid and electrolyte imbalance. Lower GI loss occurs because of sequestering of fluid in the distended bowel. Several liters of fluid may collect in the intestinal lumen, leading to a dramatic increase in lumen pressure and eventual damage to the intestinal mucosa. Peritonitis may then occur if bacteria enter the peritoneal cavity through the damaged intestinal wall. The fluid sequestered in the bowel is inaccessible to the ECF, creating a separate third space. Peritonitis also causes a shift of fluid into a temporarily inaccessible third space. Normally the peritoneum aids in the rapid transport of fluid from the peritoneal cavity to the circulation. When the peritoneum becomes damaged or inflamed, fluid and electrolytes collect in the peritoneal cavity. The loss of ECF into an inaccessible third space causes a reduction in effective circulating volume, which stimulates both thirst and release of ADH, with the retention of water. These two factors lead to the eventual development of *dilutional hyponatremia.* Upper GI loss can occur with bowel obstruction because of the increased stimulus to vomit.

## Potential Fluid, Electrolyte, and Acid-Base Disturbances with Loss of Lower Gastrointestinal Contents

1. **Hypovolemia** caused by abnormal fluid loss (see Chapter 6).
2. **Hyponatremia** caused by loss of sodium-containing fluids with inadequate electrolyte replacement; or caused by thirst and ADH-induced retention of water (see Chapter 7).
3. **Hypokalemia** caused by loss of potassium-containing fluids, combined with inadequate replacement. Hypovolemia-induced secondary hyperaldosteronism causes increased renal loss of potassium (see Chapter 8).
4. **Hypomagnesemia** caused by abnormal fluid loss (see Chapter 11). Typically hypomagnesemia occurs only with prolonged loss of GI fluids such as with ulcerative colitis.
5. **Metabolic acidosis** caused by loss of fluids rich in bicarbonate (see Chapter 15).

# Surgical Disturbances

# 19

Disturbances in fluid and electrolyte balance are common in the surgical patient because of a combination of factors that occur preoperatively, intraoperatively, and postoperatively.

## Preoperative Factors

1. **Preexisting conditions** such as diabetes mellitus, liver disease, or renal insufficiency, which may be aggravated by the stress of surgery (see Chapters 20, 22, and 24).
2. **Diagnostic procedures** such as arteriogram or intravenous pyelogram that require administration of intravenous dyes, which may cause inappropriate urinary excretion of water and electrolytes because of the osmotic diuresis effect.
3. **Administration of medications** such as steroids or diuretics, which may affect the excretion of water and electrolytes.
4. **Surgical preparations** such as enemas or laxatives, which may act to increase fluid loss from the gastrointestinal tract (see Chapter 18).
5. **Medical management of preexisting conditions.** Examples include gastric suction and gastric lavage.
6. **Preoperative fluid restriction** (i.e., nothing by mouth [NPO] after midnight). During an average 6-hour period of fluid restriction, the healthy adult patient loses approximately 300 to 500 ml of fluid as a result of normal fluid loss. Fluid loss may be increased greatly if the patient is experiencing abnormal fluid loss or fever. Because infants and toddlers have a greater relative body surface area and higher metabolic rate than adults, NPO status places them at increased risk for fluid loss. It is recommended that infants and toddlers be scheduled as first cases of the day.

# Intraoperative Factors

1. **Induction of anesthesia,** which may lead to the development of hypotension in the patient with preoperative hypovolemia because of the loss of compensatory mechanisms such as tachycardia or vasoconstriction.
2. **Abnormal blood loss** related to preoperative trauma or the surgical procedure itself.
3. **Abnormal loss of extracellular fluid (ECF) into a third space,** for example, the loss of ECF into the wall and lumen of the bowel during bowel surgery. This fluid is temporarily unavailable either to the intracellular fluid or ECF, hence it is termed *third-space fluid.* Loss of ECF also occurs when intravascular volume is lost into a nonequilibrating space, for example, bleeding into a fractured hip.
4. **Evaporative loss of fluid from the surgical wound.** This usually is of concern with large wounds and prolonged operative procedures.

NOTE: All of the above factors relate to fluid volume (see Chapter 6).

# Postoperative Factors

1. **Stress of surgery and postoperative pain,** which leads to an increased release of antidiuretic hormone (ADH) by the posterior pituitary gland and an increased release of adrenocorticotropic hormone (ACTH) by the anterior pituitary gland. Increased ADH results in retention of water by the kidneys. Excessive production may lead to the development of hyponatremia (see Chapter 7). ACTH acts on the adrenal cortex to cause an increase in the release of aldosterone and hydrocortisone. Both aldosterone and hydrocortisone lead to an increased retention of sodium and water and an increased excretion of potassium by the kidneys. The combined effects of these hormones may result in postoperative fluid retention lasting up to 48 to 72 hours (see Chapter 6).
2. **Increase in tissue catabolism** (breakdown) secondary to tissue trauma, which causes the patient to produce a greater than normal amount of water from oxidation (see Chapter 6).
3. **Reduction in effective circulating volume,** which stimulates production of ADH and aldosterone. Potential causes

include bleeding, fluid loss from the surgical wound, abnormal sequestration of fluid (i.e., third space shift), draining fistulas, gastric suction, vomiting, and increased insensible fluid loss from fever (see Chapter 6).

4. **Risk or presence of postoperative ileus,** which may restrict the patient's ability to take oral fluids and necessitate gastric suction (see Chapter 18).

5. **Hyperkalemia,** which may occur during the immediate postoperative period because of the release of intracellular potassium secondary to tissue trauma (see Chapter 8).

6. **Metabolic acidosis,** which may occur because of an abnormal production of lactic acid in the hypotensive patient who experiences tissue hypoxia (see Chapter 15).

7. **Respiratory acidosis,** which may develop as the result of inadequate ventilation secondary to respiratory depression from anesthesia or pain medication, splinting of the operative site, or restriction to bed, increasing the risk of atelectasis or pneumonia, especially in the patient with chronic obstructive pulmonary disease (see Chapter 13).

8. **Respiratory alkalosis,** which may develop initially if hypoxemia occurs as a result of postoperative pulmonary disturbance (e.g., pneumonia, pulmonary edema, pulmonary emboli) (see Chapter 14).

9. **Fluid, electrolyte, and acid-base disturbances,** which may occur with abnormal loss of GI fluids because of vomiting, diarrhea, and gastric or intestinal suctioning (see Chapter 18).

# Endocrinologic Disorders

20

## Diabetic Ketoacidosis

Diabetic ketoacidosis (DKA) is a life-threatening complication of diabetes mellitus that is characterized by hyperglycemia, dehydration, electrolyte imbalance, ketosis, and acidosis. It occurs most commonly in persons with type I insulin-dependent diabetes mellitus (IDDM) who experience illness, infection, trauma, or surgery. A relative or absolute insulin deficiency prevents the normal use of serum glucose and results in cellular starvation despite the abundance of glucose in the serum. The unmet energy requirements of the cells stimulate gluconeogenesis and glycogen conversion in the liver and trigger the release of catabolic stress hormones, which act to elevate the serum glucose even further. The body is forced to break down its fat and protein stores to meet the energy requirements of cell metabolism. The rate of breakdown exceeds the body's ability to use these alternate energy sources, however, and ketone bodies accumulate in the blood. Ketones cause the blood pH level to drop, which results in the potential for profound metabolic ketoacidosis. Hyperglycemia results in increased serum osmolality.

Glucose and ketones not reabsorbed by the renal tubule cause an osmotic diuresis, with losses of sodium, potassium, phosphorus, magnesium, and body water, which can lead to severe dehydration and hypovolemic shock. Despite significant loss of potassium in the urine, the patient initially may present with normal or elevated plasma potassium because of the dramatic shift of potassium out of the cells secondary to insulin deficiency, acidosis, and tissue catabolism. Increased blood viscosity and platelet aggregation can result in thromboembolism. Dehydration also decreases tissue perfusion, and the resulting lactic acid waste products exacerbate the existing acidosis. The lowered pH level stimulates the respiratory center, producing the deep, rapid respirations known as

Kussmaul's respirations. The large amount of ketones lends a fruity or acetone odor to the breath. If not treated promptly, elevated serum osmolality, acidosis, and dehydration depress consciousness to the point of coma. Death can result from hypovolemia or profound central nervous system (CNS) depression.

## Potential Fluid, Electrolyte, and Acid-Base Disturbances

1. **Fluid volume deficit** caused by polyuria secondary to hyperglycemia and ketonemia. Initially, hypovolemia is treated with isotonic saline (0.9% NaCl) administered at a rapid rate. Subsequent volume replacement is with 0.45% NaCl solution, which more closely approximates the fluid loss. Once the blood glucose level falls to 250 to 300 mg/dl, dextrose-containing solutions are used (e.g., 5% dextrose in 0.45% NaCl or 5% dextrose in 0.225% NaCl).

2. **Hyponatremia** (initially) caused by the osmotic shift of water out of the cells (pseudohyponatremia) and caused by the loss of sodium in the urine (see Chapter 7).

3. **Hypernatremia** caused by dehydration secondary to osmotic diuresis with the loss of free water (i.e., water is lost in excess of electrolytes). Hypernatremia is corrected with administration of hypotonic intravenous (IV) fluids (see Chapter 7).

4. **Hyperkalemia** (initially) caused by movement of potassium out of the cell secondary to tissue catabolism, acidosis, and insulin deficiency (see Chapter 8).

5. **Hyperphosphatemia** (initially) caused by the movement of phosphorus out of the cell secondary to tissue catabolism (see Chapter 10).

6. **Hypokalemia** caused by the loss of potassium secondary to osmotic diuresis and the movement of potassium back into the cell, occurring with the administration of insulin and correction of acidosis. Potassium levels may drop precipitously with treatment of DKA, requiring frequent monitoring and aggressive potassium replacement (see Chapter 8).

7. **Hypophosphatemia and hypomagnesemia** caused by the loss of these electrolytes secondary to osmotic diuresis and repair of the tissue with treatment. Hypophosphatemia is corrected by replacing a portion of the potassium deficit with potassium phosphate (see Chapters 10 and 11).

8. **Metabolic acidosis** occurring with the abnormal production of ketoacids and lactic acid. Metabolic acidosis usually reverses with the administration of insulin and fluids. Severe acidosis, however, may require treatment with IV sodium bicarbonate (see Chapter 15).

9. **Hypochloremia** may be present initially because of the loss of chloride in the urine and the movement of water out of the cells. Hyperchloremia may occur with treatment because of administration of isotonic NaCl solution, which contains chloride in a concentration exceeding the plasma chloride level.

# Hyperosmolar Hyperglycemic Nonketotic Syndrome

Hyperosmolar hyperglycemic nonketotic (HHNK) syndrome is a life-threatening emergency characterized by severe hyperglycemia (blood glucose levels exceed 600 mg/dl and may be as high as 2000 mg/dl) with the absence of significant ketonemia. As with DKA, hyperglycemia causes an osmotic diuresis with loss of electrolytes, including sodium, chloride, potassium, magnesium, and phosphorus. The diuresis is hypotonic in relation to the electrolytes (i.e., water is lost in excess of sodium and other electrolytes). The combination of hypotonic fluid loss and hyperglycemia leads to serum hyperosmolality. In turn, increased serum osmolality causes a shift of water out of the cells. The net result is a loss of both intracellular fluid (ICF) and extracellular fluid (ECF), with individuals losing up to 25% of their total body water. Neurologic deficits (i.e., slowed mentation, confusion, seizures, or coma) occur as a result of the altered CNS cell function secondary to cell shrinkage.

As extracellular volume decreases, the blood becomes more viscous and its flow is impeded. Thromboemboli are common because of increased blood viscosity, enhanced platelet aggregation and adhesiveness, and patient immobility. Cardiac workload is increased and may lead to myocardial infarction. Renal blood flow is decreased, potentially resulting in renal impairment or failure. Cerebrovascular accident may result from thromboemboli or decreased cerebral perfusion. These severe complications, in addition to the initial precipitating disorder, have contributed to a mortality rate of 10% to 25%.

The onset of HHNK syndrome is often insidious and classically occurs in the older individual with non–insulin-dependent diabetes who has a concomitant reduction in renal function. It is typically precipitated by some form of stress (e.g., infection, trauma, surgery) that increases the release of hormones (i.e., catecholamines, glucagon, and cortisol), which raises blood glucose levels. The combination of hypovolemia and decreased renal function ultimately results in a rapid rise in blood glucose secondary to decreased urinary excretion of glucose. The mechanism responsible for the absence of elevated ketones is not fully understood, although it has been suggested that individuals who develop HHNK syndrome still produce enough insulin to maintain normal fat metabolism but which is insufficient for normal glucose use. The absence of ketoacidosis and the slow onset of vague neurologic symptoms in the older adult often result in HHNK syndrome initially being misdiagnosed as a primary neurologic disorder. See Table 20-1 for a comparison of DKA and HHNK syndrome.

## Potential Fluid, Electrolyte, and Acid-Base Disturbances

1. **Fluid volume deficit** caused by hyperglycemia-induced osmotic diuresis. Hypovolemia is treated with either isotonic saline (0.9% NaCl) or 0.45% saline (see Chapter 6).
2. **Hyponatremia** may be present initially because of the osmotic shift of water out of the cells (pseudohyponatremia). The presence of hypertriglyceridemia may also contribute to pseudohyponatremia. In fact, glucose-induced osmotic diuresis causes a hypotonic fluid loss, with water being lost in excess of sodium. If the plasma sodium on admission is normal or elevated, a massive water loss has occurred (see Chapter 7).
3. **Hypokalemia** caused by increased urinary losses secondary to osmotic diuresis (see Chapter 8).
4. **Hypophosphatemia** caused by increased urinary losses secondary to osmotic diuresis. Hypokalemia and hypophosphatemia are treated with a combination of IV potassium chloride and potassium phosphate (see Chapter 10).
5. **Hypomagnesemia** caused by increased urinary losses secondary to osmotic diuresis (see Chapter 11).
6. **Metabolic acidosis** caused by increased production and retention of lactic acid secondary to hypovolemia with tissue hypoxia. Acidosis usually resolves with treatment (insulin

Table 20-1    Comparison of diabetic ketoacidosis (DKA) and hyperosmolar hyperglycemic nonketotic (HHNK) syndrome

| Criterion | DKA | HHNK |
|---|---|---|
| Diabetes type | Usually IDDM (type I) | Usually NIDDM (type II) |
| Typical age group | Any age | Usually >50 yr |
| Signs and symptoms | Polyuria, polydipsia, polyphagia, weakness, orthostatic hypotension, lethargy, changes in LOC, fatigue, nausea, vomiting, abdominal pain | Same as DKA, but slower onset and, very commonly, neurologic symptoms predominate |
| Physical assessment | Dry and flushed skin, poor skin turgor, dry mucous membranes, decreased BP, tachycardia, altered LOC (irritability, lethargy, coma), Kussmaul's respirations, fruity odor to the breath | Same as DKA, but no Kussmaul's respirations or fruity odor to the breath; instead, occurrence of tachypnea with shallow respirations |
| History and risk factors | Recent stressors such as surgery, trauma, infection, MI; insufficient exogenous insulin; undiagnosed type I diabetes mellitus | Undiagnosed type II diabetes mellitus; recent stressors such as surgery, trauma, pancreatitis, MI, infection; high-caloric enteral or parenteral feedings in a compromised patient; use of diabetogenic drugs (e.g., phenytoin, thiazide diuretics, thyroid preparations, mannitol, corticosteroids, sympathomimetics) |

| | | |
|---|---|---|
| Monitoring parameters | *ECG:* Dysrhythmias associated with hyperkalemia: peaked T waves, widened QRS complex, prolonged PR interval, flattened or absent P wave. Hypokalemia ($K^+$ <3 mEq/L), which may produce depressed ST segments, flat or inverted T waves, or increased ventricular dysrhythmias | ECG evidence of hypokalemia as listed with DKA<br>*Hemodynamic measurements:* CVP >3 mm Hg below patient's baseline; PADP and PAWP >4 mm Hg below patient's baseline |
| Diagnostic tests | *Serum glucose:* 200-800 mg/dl | 800-2000 mg/dl |
| | *Serum acetone:* positive | Usually absent |
| | *Urine glucose:* positive | Positive |
| | *Urine acetone:* "large" | Negative |
| | *Serum osmolality:* 300-350 mOsm/L | >350 mOsm/L |
| | *Bicarbonate:* <15 mEq/L | Normal or slightly decreased if mild acidosis present |
| | *Serum pH:* <7.2 | Normal or mildly acidotic (pH <7.4) |
| | *Serum potassium:* normal or elevated >5 mEq/L initially and then decreased | Normal or <3.5 mEq/L |

From Horne MM: Endocrinologic dysfunctions. In Swearingen PL, Keen JH, editors: *Manual of critical care nursing: nursing interventions and collaborative management,* ed 3, St Louis, 1995, Mosby.

*IDDM,* Insulin-dependent diabetes mellitus; *NIDDM,* non–insulin-dependent diabetes mellitus; *LOC,* level of consciousness; *BP,* blood pressure; *MI,* myocardial infarction; *CVP,* central venous pressure; *PADP,* pulmonary artery diastolic pressure; *PAWP,* pulmonary artery wedge pressure.

*Continued*

**Table 20-1**   Comparison of diabetic ketoacidosis (DKA) and hyperosmolar hyperglycemic nonketotic (HHNK) syndrome—cont'd

| Criterion | DKA | HHNK |
|---|---|---|
| | *Serum sodium:* elevated, normal, or low | Elevated, normal, or low |
| | *Serum Hct:* elevated because of osmotic diuresis with hemoconcentration | Elevated because of hemoconcentration |
| | *BUN:* elevated >20 mg/dl | Elevated |
| | *Serum creatinine:* >1.5 mg/dl | Elevated |
| | *Serum phosphorus, magnesium, chloride:* decreased | Decreased |
| | *WBC:* elevated, even in the absence of infection | Normal unless infection present |
| Onset | Hours to days | Days to weeks |
| Mortality rate | <10% | 10%-25% as a result of age group and complications such as CVA, thrombosis, renal failure |

*CVA,* Cerebrovascular accident.

and fluids) but may be treated with IV sodium bicarbonate if it is severe (see Chapter 15).

# Diabetes Insipidus

Diabetes Insipidus (DI) is caused by either a deficiency in the synthesis or release of antidiuretic hormone (ADH) from the posterior pituitary gland (neurogenic or central DI) or a decrease in kidney responsiveness to ADH (nephrogenic DI), resulting in decreased water absorption by the renal tubules. Central DI may be idiopathic or may occur as a result of cerebral tumor, trauma, or hypoperfusion and resolves with the administration of vasopressin (Table 20-2). In contrast, nephrogenic DI responds poorly to vasopressin and may be caused by a wide variety of medications and disorders, including electrolyte imbalance (i.e., hypokalemia or hypocalcemia).

Regardless of the cause, the individual with DI excretes large volumes of extremely dilute urine. As with diabetes mellitus, the cardinal symptoms of DI are polyuria and polydipsia. These remain the only symptoms as long as these individuals are able to drink and satisfy their thirst, thereby maintaining fluid volume. If the person is unable to access adequate amounts of water (e.g., an infant with congenital DI or the adult who is neurologically impaired), abnormal water loss will result in rapidly decreased ECF volume and increased serum sodium and osmolality. Without treatment, severe ECF and ICF dehydration, hypotension, and shock can occur. Decreased cerebral perfusion and increased serum osmolality will produce neurologic symptoms ranging from confusion, restlessness, and irritability to seizures and coma. The severity of and prognosis for DI vary with its cause. The onset may be sudden and dramatic with cerebral trauma, or it can be gradual, as with tumors or infiltrative disease.

# Potential Fluid, Electrolyte, and Acid-Base Disturbances

1. **Fluid volume deficit** caused by decreased water reabsorption by the renal tubule secondary to decreased ADH production or effectiveness. It is treated with hypotonic fluid replacement and correction of the cause (see Chapter 6).

2. **Hypernatremia** caused by increased free water loss secondary to decreased renal reabsorption of water. Hypernatremia also is corrected by hypotonic fluid replacement. Ironically, nephrogenic DI can be treated with diuretics such as thiazide

**Table 20-2** Vasopressin preparations

| Generic Name | Trade Name | Onset | Duration | Usual Dosage | Advantages/Disadvantages | Comments |
|---|---|---|---|---|---|---|
| **Nasal** | | | | | | |
| Vasopressin | Pitressin | Within 1 hour | 4-8 hours | 5-10 U bid-tid | Action decreased by nasal congestion/discharge or atrophy of nasal mucosa | Administer by spray, cotton pledget, or dropper; used for chronic DI management |
| Desmopressin acetate | DDAVP | Within 1 hour | 8-20 hours | 0.1-0.4 ml qd in 1-3 doses (10-40 µg) | See above | See above; stored in refrigerator at 4°C (39.2°F) |
| Lypressin | Diapid | Within 1 hour | 3-8 hours | 7-14 µg qid | See above | See above; stored at <40°C (100°F) |

| | | | | | |
|---|---|---|---|---|---|
| **Subcutaneous** | | | | | |
| Vasopressin | Pitressin | ½-1 hour | 2-8 hours | 0.25-0.5 ml (5-10 U) q3-4h prn for increased thirst or urine output | Typically used in acute care setting and for emergency management Kept refrigerated at 4°C (39.2°F) |
| Desmopressin acetate | DDAVP, Stimate | Within ½ hour | 1½-4 hours | 0.5-1 ml (2-4 µg) qd in 2 divided doses | |
| **Intramuscular** | | | | | |
| Vasopressin tannate in oil | Pitressin tannate in oil | Within 1-2 hours | 36-48 hours | 0.3-1 ml (1.5-5 U) q2-3d for increased thirst or increased urine output | Longer duration of action/ slower absorption than SC route; response cumulative over 2-3 days Stored at 13°-18°C (55°-65°F) Shake well before withdrawing from vial; can warm solution by immersing vial in warm water |

*Continued*

From Horne MM: Endocrinologic dysfunctions. In Swearingen PL, Keen JH, editors: *Manual of critical care nursing: nursing interventions and collaborative management*, ed 3, St Louis, 1995, Mosby.

*DI*, Diabetes insipidus; *DDAVP*, 1-deamino-8-D-arginine vasopressin.

**Table 20-2** Vasopressin preparations—cont'd

| Generic Name | Trade Name | Onset | Duration | Usual Dosage | Advantages/ Disadvantages | Comments |
|---|---|---|---|---|---|---|
| Vasopressin tannate | Pitressin tannate | ½-1 hour | 2-8 hours | 0.25-0.5 ml (5-10 U) q3-4h for increased thirst or increased urine output | Longer duration of action, which makes intramuscular forms more desirable for chronic management | |
| Intravenous Desmopressin acetate | DDAVP | Within ½ hour | 1½-4 hours | 0.5-1 ml (2-4 µg) qd in 2 divided doses | Not for home use | Keep refrigerated at 4°C (39.2°F); dilute in 10-50 ml 0.9% NaCl and infuse over 15-30 minutes |

that block the kidneys' ability to excrete free water (see Chapter 7).

# Syndrome of Inappropriate Secretion of Antidiuretic Hormone

Syndrome of inappropriate secretion of antidiuretic hormone (SIADH) develops as the result of excessive levels of circulating ADH. The causes of SIADH fall into one of three categories: (1) excessive production or release of ADH secondary to CNS disorders such as meningitis or increased intracranial pressure; (2) respiratory disorders such as infections and lesions, which increase the release of ADH by an unknown mechanism; or (3) ectopic ADH secretion of malignant tumors, particularly oat cell carcinoma of the lung. In the presence of increased ADH, water that normally would be excreted in the urine is *inappropriately* reabsorbed and returned to the circulation, diluting the serum sodium and decreasing serum osmolality. ECF volume expansion increases glomerular filtration and decreases the release of aldosterone, both of which act to increase urinary excretion of sodium, further reducing the serum sodium level. As the serum sodium level decreases, an osmotic gradient is created that favors an ICF shift. Increased ICF in the brain can result in cerebral edema with altered neurologic function and, ultimately, death if the condition is not treated.

SIADH typically is diagnosed on the basis of laboratory findings and patient history. Classic laboratory findings include serum hyponatremia and hypoosmolality, combined with inappropriately high urine sodium and osmolality. Treatment is aimed at correcting the primary problem, limiting water intake, and administering sodium. Medications such as lithium or demeclocycline, which inhibit the action of ADH on the renal tubule, may also be used.

## Potential Fluid, Electrolyte and Acid-Base Disturbances

1. **Hyponatremia** caused by excessive retention of water and continued urinary loss of sodium (see Chapter 7).
2. **Hypervolemia** caused by retention of water with cellular volume expansion (see Chapter 6). NOTE: ECF volume expansion usually is minimized because of the decreased stimulus to aldosterone and increased stimulus to atrial natriuretic factor.

## Acute Adrenal Insufficiency

Adrenal insufficiency (decreased production of adrenocortical hormones) occurs as a result of either dysfunction of the adrenal glands (primary) or inadequate stimulation of the adrenal glands by the anterior pituitary (secondary). Conditions associated with primary adrenal insufficiency include autoimmune disease, infection, bilateral adrenal hemorrhage, bilateral adrenalectomy, tumor invasion, and enzymatic deficiencies. A decrease in the production of adrenocortical hormones because of a reduction in functioning adrenal tissue is also termed *Addison's disease.* Secondary adrenal insufficiency is associated with exogenous steroid administration and destruction of the pituitary gland by tumors, infarcts, trauma, surgery, or infection.

Acute adrenal insufficiency (Addisonian crisis) is a life-threatening condition characterized by severe fluid and electrolyte imbalances related to both mineralocorticoid and glucocorticoid deficiencies. Mineralocorticoid (aldosterone) deficiency results in large urinary losses of sodium and water with the development of hyponatremia and hypovolemia. In addition, hyperkalemia and metabolic acidosis can develop as the result of decreased urinary excretion of potassium and hydrogen. Glucocorticoid (cortisol) deficiency intensifies the clinical effects of hypovolemia by causing a decrease in vascular tone and decreased vascular response to catecholamines (epinephrine and norepinephrine). Cortisol depletion also may cause hypoglycemia because of the body's inability to maintain blood glucose levels in the fasting state. Severe hypotension, shock, and eventually death will occur without adequate parenteral adrenocortical hormone and fluid replacement. In patients with chronic insufficiency, acute crises may be prevented by tripling replacement hormone doses during periods of stress.

## Potential Fluid, Electrolyte, and Acid-Base Disturbances

1. **Hypovolemia** caused by decreased reabsorption of sodium and water by the renal tubule secondary to the lack of aldosterone. It is treated with IV isotonic (0.9%) saline solution and IV hydrocortisone (see Chapter 6).
2. **Hyperkalemia** caused by decreased secretion and excretion of potassium by the renal tubule secondary to the lack of aldosterone. Hyperkalemia is treated with kayexalate (see Chapter 8).

3. **Metabolic acidosis,** termed *Type 4 renal tubular acidosis,* caused by decreased secretion and excretion of hydrogen by the renal tubule secondary to the lack of aldosterone. Hyperkalemia may contribute to the development of metabolic acidosis because it impairs $NH_4$ production (see Chapter 15).

4. **Hyponatremia,** which may occur in chronic primary adrenocortical insufficiency because of hypovolemia-induced release of ADH with the retention of free water (see Chapter 7).

# Cardiac Disorders 21

## Congestive Heart Failure and Pulmonary Edema

Congestive heart failure (CHF) develops when the heart is unable to maintain a cardiac output sufficient to meet the metabolic needs of the tissues. Causes of CHF include coronary artery disease, hypertension, cardiomyopathy, and valvular disease. As the heart fails and the cardiac output drops, there is a reduction in effective circulating volume (ECV) with poor renal blood flow. This results in a reduction in the load of sodium and water filtered by the kidneys and stimulates the release of renin. Renin causes an increase in angiotensin II, a potent vasoconstrictor that increases systemic vascular resistance and the workload of the heart (afterload). Increased angiotensin II, in turn, leads to an increase in aldosterone, with retention of sodium and water by the kidneys and an increase in vascular volume (preload). Decreased ECV also stimulates the release of antidiuretic hormone (ADH), causing further retention of water by the kidneys. Because the diseased heart is unable to circulate this increased volume, the pressure within the venous circuit increases and edema develops.

When the left side of the heart is unable to pump the blood returning from the lungs into systemic circulation, the hydrostatic pressure within the pulmonary circulation increases. If the hydrostatic pressure exceeds the pulmonary oncotic pressure, fluid leaks into the pulmonary interstitium. This results in pulmonary edema with impairment of oxygen exchange. Right ventricular failure usually occurs secondary to left ventricular failure (the right heart must work harder as the pressure in the pulmonary vasculature increases), but may occur independently in conditions such as cor pulmonale. When the right side of the heart fails, there is a backup in the venous circuit, with congestion of blood in body organs (e.g., liver and spleen) and edema formation.

## Potential Fluid, Electrolyte, and Acid-Base Disturbances

1. **Fluid volume excess,** as evidenced by peripheral and pulmonary edema, caused by increased secretion of aldosterone and ADH. It is treated with diuretics and fluid and sodium restriction. Inotropic agents and vasodilators are administered to improve cardiac function (see Chapter 6).
2. **Hyponatremia** caused by increased secretion of ADH (remember ADH affects water retention only, whereas aldosterone causes retention of both sodium and water). Hyponatremia resolves with fluid restriction and correction of the primary problem (see Chapter 7).
3. **Hypokalemia** caused by the use of potassium-wasting diuretics (e.g., furosemide). Furosemide commonly is used in the treatment of acute pulmonary edema because of its potent and rapid diuretic action when administered intravenously (IV) and its direct vasodilatory effect, which reduces preload (see Chapter 8).
4. **Respiratory alkalosis** may occur in pulmonary edema because of hypoxemia-induced hyperventilation (see Chapter 14).
5. **Respiratory acidosis** may develop if pulmonary edema is so severe that carbon dioxide retention occurs with hypoxemia (see Chapter 13).
6. **Metabolic acidosis** may develop in individuals in cardiogenic shock because of increased production of lactic acid by hypoxic tissues and decreased excretion of acids by the kidney (see Chapter 15).

## Cardiogenic Shock

Shock is a state in which blood flow to peripheral tissue is inadequate for sustaining life. Usually cardiogenic shock is caused by a massive myocardial infarction that renders 40% or more of the myocardium dysfunctional secondary to necrosis or ischemia. As a result, cardiac output is reduced and all tissues suffer from inadequate perfusion. With decreased perfusion to the heart, coronary flow is reduced, impairing cardiac function, which further decreases cardiac output.

The first stage of shock is characterized by increased sympathetic discharge as the baroreceptors at the carotid sinus and aortic arch are stimulated by the drop in blood pressure. The release of epinephrine and norepinephrine is a compensatory mechanism that increases cardiac output by increasing the heart rate and contractility of the uninjured myocardium. Vasoconstriction, a mechanism that increases blood pressure, also occurs. The second or middle stage of shock is characterized by decreased perfusion to the brain, kidneys, and heart. Lactate and pyruvic acid accumulate in the tissues, and metabolic acidosis occurs secondary to anaerobic metabolism. In the late stage of shock, which is usually irreversible, compensatory mechanisms become ineffective, and multiple organ failure occurs.

## Potential Fluid, Electrolyte, and Acid-Base Disturbances

1. **Fluid volume deficit** may be present because of prior diuretic therapy with potent diuretics (e.g., furosemide) (see Chapter 6).
2. **Fluid volume excess** may be present or develop because of stimulation of the renin-angiotensin system, resulting in retention of sodium and water. Overly aggressive fluid therapy may contribute. Volume imbalances will resolve with improved cardiac function (see Chapter 6).
3. **Hyponatremia** may be present secondary to an increase in the release of ADH, resulting in retention of water (see Chapter 7).
4. **Metabolic acidosis** occurring with accumulation of lactate and pyruvic acid in the tissues secondary to decreased tissue perfusion. Severe metabolic acidosis may require treatment with IV sodium bicarbonate (see Chapter 15).
5. **If shock is prolonged,** the individual may develop acute tubular necrosis, which can lead to multiple fluid and electrolyte disturbances (see Chapter 22).

# Renal Failure

22

Because the kidneys are the primary regulators of fluid and electrolyte balance, renal failure (either acute or chronic) may lead to a myriad of disturbances in fluid and electrolyte balance. This is easy to appreciate after reviewing the normal functions of the kidneys (see the box on p. 222).

Acute renal failure (ARF) is a sudden loss of renal function that may or may not be accompanied by oliguria. The kidneys lose the ability to maintain biochemical homeostasis, causing retention of metabolic waste and dramatic alterations in fluid, electrolyte, and acid-base balance. Although the alteration in renal function usually is reversible, ARF is associated with an overall mortality rate as high as 40%. However, the mortality rate varies greatly with the etiology of ARF, the patient's age, and preexisting medical problems.

The causes of ARF are classified according to etiology as prerenal, intrarenal, and postrenal (see the box on p. 223). A decrease in renal function secondary to decreased renal perfusion but without renal parenchymal damage is termed *prerenal failure.* Causes of prerenal failure include fluid volume deficit, shock, and decreased cardiac function. If hypoperfusion has not been prolonged, restoration of renal perfusion will restore normal renal function. A reduction in urine output that occurs because of obstruction to urine flow is termed *postrenal* or *postobstructive failure.* Conditions causing postrenal failure include neurogenic bladder, tumors, and urethral strictures. Early detection of prerenal and postrenal failure is essential because, if prolonged, they can lead to parenchymal damage.

The most common cause of *intrarenal* or *intrinsic failure,* renal failure that develops secondary to renal parenchymal damage, is acute tubular necrosis (ATN). Although typically associated with prolonged ischemia (prerenal failure) or exposure to nephrotoxins, ATN also can occur after transfusion reactions, crushing injuries, or

## Functions of the Kidney

- Regulation of water and electrolyte balance. The kidneys play an important role in the regulation of sodium ion ($Na^+$), potassium ion ($K^+$), calcium ion ($Ca^{2+}$), magnesium ion ($Mg^{2+}$), hydrogen ion ($H^+$), chloride ion ($Cl^-$), phosphate ion ($PO_4^{3-}$), and bicarbonate ion ($HCO_3^-$).
- Maintenance of acid-base balance through the excretion of $H^+$ and the regeneration of $HCO_3^-$. As each hydrogen ion is moved into the renal tubule to be excreted, a bicarbonate ion is generated and returned to the extracellular fluid.
- Excretion of metabolic wastes (i.e., urea, uric acid, creatinine, unknown toxins).
- Excretion of foreign substances (i.e., medications, poisons, food additives).
- Production of the following:

   —*Renin:* Helps regulate vascular volume and blood pressure through the regulation of $Na^+$ and water.

   —*Erythropoietin:* Released in response to a low oxygen level in the renal cells; it stimulates the production of red blood cells by the bone marrow.

   —*Active form of vitamin D:* Increases the intestinal absorption of calcium, phosphorus, and magnesium; increases bone resorption (movement out) of calcium and phosphorus; and increases the reabsorption (saving) of calcium and phosphorus by the kidney. The net result is that of helping maintain normal calcium, phosphorus, and magnesium levels.

   —*Prostaglandins:* Primarily vasodilating substances, they affect blood flow to and within the kidney and increase kidney responsiveness to the effects of antidiuretic hormone and aldosterone.

septic abortions. The clinical course of ATN is divided into three phases: oliguric (lasting approximately 7 to 21 days); diuretic (lasting 7 to 14 days); and recovery (which can continue for 3 to 12 months). Causes of intrarenal failure other than ATN include acute glomerulonephritis and malignant hypertension. See the box on p. 225 for a list of drugs that require dosage modification for patients with ARF.

## Causes of Acute Renal Failure

| Prerenal (Decreased Renal Perfusion) | Intrarenal (Parenchymal Damage; Acute Tubular Necrosis) | Postrenal (Obstruction) |
|---|---|---|
| **Fluid Volume Deficit** | **Nephrotoxic Agents** | **Calculi** |
| ▪ GI losses | ▪ Antibiotics (aminoglycosides, sulfonamides, methicillin) | **Tumor** |
| ▪ Hemorrhage | ▪ Diuretics (e.g., furosemide) | **Benign Prostate Hypertrophy** |
| ▪ Third-space (interstitial) losses (burns, peritonitis) | ▪ Contrast media | **Necrotizing Papillitis** |
| ▪ Dehydration from diuretic use | ▪ Heavy metals (lead, gold, mercury) | **Urethral Strictures** |
| | ▪ Organic solvents (carbon tetrachloride, ethylene glycol) | |
| **Hepatorenal Syndrome** | | **Blood Clots** |
| **Edema-Forming Conditions** | **Infection (Gram-Negative Sepsis), Pancreatitis, Peritonitis** | **Retroperitoneal Fibrosis** |
| ▪ Congestive heart failure | | |
| ▪ Cirrhosis | **Transfusion Reaction (Hemolysis)** | **Neurogenic Bladder** |
| ▪ Nephrotic syndrome | | |

*Continued*

*GI,* Gastrointestinal.

## Causes of Acute Renal Failure—cont'd

| Prerenal (Decreased Renal Perfusion) | Intrarenal (Parenchymal Damage; Acute Tubular Necrosis) | Postrenal (Obstruction) |
|---|---|---|
| **Renal Vascular Disorders**<br>■ Renal artery stenosis<br>■ Renal artery thrombosis<br>■ Renal vein thrombosis | **Rhabdomyolysis with Myoglobinuria (Severe Muscle Injury)**<br>■ Trauma (crush injuries)<br>■ Exertion<br>■ Seizures<br>■ Drug-related: heroin, barbiturates, intravenous amphetamines<br><br>**Glomerular Diseases**<br>■ Poststreptococcal glomerulonephritis<br>■ IgA nephropathy (e.g., Berger's disease)<br>■ Lupus glomerulonephritis<br>■ Serum sickness<br>■ Acute interstitial nephritis (drug induced)<br><br>**Ischemic Injury (Prolonged Prerenal)** | |

## Drugs that Require Dosage Modification in Renal Failure

| Antimicrobials | Cardiovascular Agents | Analgesics | Sedatives | Miscellaneous | Drugs to Avoid |
|---|---|---|---|---|---|
| Amikacin | Digoxin | Meperidine | Phenobarbital | Insulin | Tetracycline |
| Gentamicin | Procainamide | Methadone | Meprobamate | Cimetidine | Nitrofurantoin |
| Kanamycin | Guanethidine | | | Clofibrate | Spironolactone |
| Tobramycin | | | | | Amiloride |
| Amphotericin B | | | | | Aspirin |
| Vancomycin | | | | | Lithium carbonate |
| Lincomycin | | | | | Cisplatin |
| Sulfonamides | | | | | Nonsteroidal anti- |
| Ethambutol | | | | | inflammatory |
| Penicillins | | | | | agents |
| | | | | | Magnesium- |
| | | | | | containing |
| | | | | | medications |

Chronic renal failure (CRF) is a progressive, irreversible loss of renal function that develops over months to years. Eventually it can progress to end-stage renal disease (ESRD), at which time renal replacement therapy (dialysis or transplantation) is required to sustain life. Before ESRD occurs, the individual with CRF can lead a relatively normal life managed by diet and medications. The length of this period varies, depending on the cause of renal failure and the patient's level of renal function at the time of diagnosis.

There are many causes of CRF, some of the most common being glomerulonephritis, diabetes mellitus, hypertension, and polycystic kidney disease. Regardless of the cause, the clinical presentation of CRF, particularly as the individual approaches ESRD, is similar. Retention of nitrogenous wastes and accompanying fluid and electrolyte imbalances adversely affect all body systems. Alterations in neuromuscular, cardiovascular, and gastrointestinal function are common. Renal osteodystrophy is an early and frequent complication. These collective manifestations of CRF are termed *uremia.*

## Potential Fluid, Electrolyte, and Acid-Base Disturbances

1. **Hypervolemia** caused by anuria or oliguria. It is treated with fluid restriction, diuretics, and, if necessary, dialysis (see Figures 22-1 and 22-2 for depictions of dialysis and see Chapter 6).

2. **Hypovolemia** during the diuretic phase of ARF because of excretion of large volumes of hypotonic urine, combined with existing fluid restriction. Hypovolemia also may occur in postrenal failure after release of the obstruction (postobstructive diuresis). Hypovolemia may be the precipitating event in prerenal failure (see the box on p. 223 and see Chapter 6).

3. **Hyponatremia** caused by excessive consumption or administration of hypotonic fluids (see Chapter 7).

4. **Hyperkalemia** caused by the kidneys' inability to excrete potassium and increased tissue catabolism with the release of intracellular potassium. Hyperkalemia is managed by a combination of dietary restrictions and removal via cation exchange resins or dialysis. Acute, life-threatening hyperkalemia may be temporarily corrected by the administration of glucose and insulin or sodium bicarbonate (see Chapter 8).

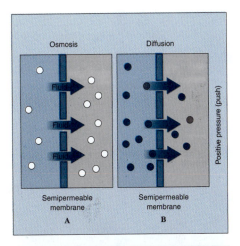

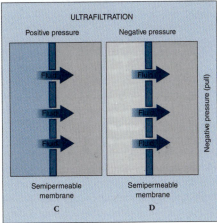

## Figure 22-1

Dialysis is based on principles of osmosis **(A)**, diffusion, and **(B)** ultrafiltration. Ultrafiltration occurs when either positive pressure **(C)** or negative pressure **(D)** is placed on the system. Ultrafiltration can be maximized by exerting positive and negative pressure on the system simultaneously.

(From Phipps WJ et al: *Medical-surgical nursing: concepts and clinical practice,* ed 5, St Louis, 1995, Mosby.)

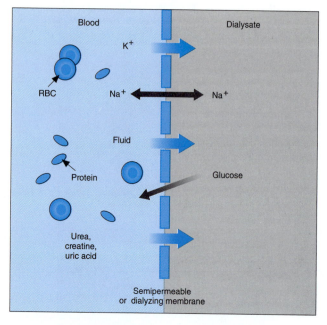

Figure 22-2
Osmosis and diffusion in dialysis. Net movement of major particles and fluid is illustrated.
(From Phipps WJ et al: *Medical-surgical nursing: concepts and clinical practice,* ed 5, St Louis, 1995, Mosby.)

5. **Hypokalemia** during the diuretic phase of ARF, especially in the potassium-restricted patient (see Chapter 8).

6. **Hyperphosphatemia** caused by the kidneys' inability to excrete phosphorus. It is treated by limiting dietary intake of high-phosphorus foods and administration of phosphorus-binding antacids (see Chapter 10).

7. **Hypocalcemia** caused by decreased levels of the metabolically active form of vitamin D, hyperphosphatemia (remember that calcium and phosphorus have a reciprocal relationship: as one increases, the other tends to decrease), skeletal resistance to PTH (the hormone released by the parathyroid gland in response to a low serum calcium level), and hypoalbuminemia. Treatment begins with regu-

lation of phosphorus via calcium carbonate antacids. Later vitamin D replacement and additional calcium supplements may be necessary (see Chapter 9).

8. **Hypermagnesemia** caused by the kidneys' inability to excrete magnesium. Hypermagnesemia usually can be prevented by avoiding magnesium-containing medications and supplements (see Chapter 11).

9. **Metabolic acidosis** caused by the kidneys' inability to excrete the body's daily load of nonvolatile acid. Limiting dietary intake of protein and preventing tissue catabolism help minimize acidosis. Dialysis provides some buffer replacement through the addition of bicarbonate or acetate to the dialysate (see Figures 22-1 and 22-2 for depictions of dialysis and see Chapter 15).

# Acute Pancreatitis

23

Acute pancreatitis is a potentially life-threatening condition caused by abnormal activation of pancreatic enzymes. A variety of conditions are associated with pancreatitis, including trauma and infection; however, the most common are chronic alcoholism and biliary tract disease (see the box on p. 231). Although the exact pathogenesis is unknown, injury to acinar cells results in the release and activation of pancreatic enzymes, causing autodigestion of the gland. Damage to the pancreas can range from acute edema to necrosis and hemorrhage. The individual with acute pancreatitis experiences acute abdominal pain and tenderness that may be precipitated by a meal or heavy alcohol intake. Nausea, weakness, ileus, diaphoresis, tachycardia, and hypotension often are present. Laboratory findings include elevated levels of serum amylase, serum lipase, and urine amylase and decreased levels of serum calcium and serum albumin.

Several potentially severe complications may accompany acute pancreatitis. The most common complication is intravascular fluid volume deficit secondary to loss of fluid into the interstitium and retroperitoneum. Release of vasoactive amines results in increased capillary permeability, vasodilation, and depressed myocardial function. Hypoalbuminemia and hemorrhage from rupture of necrotic pancreatic vessels also may contribute to intravascular volume loss. Hypovolemia and hypotension, in turn, can lead to the development of prerenal acute renal failure (ARF) and shock. Other severe complications include tetany secondary to severe hypocalcemia, respiratory failure, and rupture of abscessed pancreatic pseudocytes.

## Potential Fluid, Electrolyte, and Acid-Base Disturbances

1. **Fluid volume deficit** caused by loss of fluid into the interstitium and retroperitoneum, vomiting, gastric suction, diarrhea, dia-

## Precipitating Factors for Acute Pancreatitis

### Mechanical Blockage of Pancreatic Ducts

- Biliary tract disease (e.g., gallstones)
- Structural abnormalities (e.g., pancreas divisum)

### Toxic and Metabolic Factors

- Alcohol
- Hypertriglyceridemia
- Hypercalcemia (e.g., hyperparathyroidism)

### Infection

### Trauma

- External
- Surgical
- Iatrogenic

### Ischemia

- Prolonged/severe shock
- Vasculitis

### Tumors

### Drugs

- Nonsteroidal antiinflammatory drugs
- Estrogens
- Corticosteroids
- Sulfonamides

From Keen JH: Gastrointestinal dysfunctions. In Swearingen PL, Keen JH, editors: *Manual of critical care nursing: nursing interventions and collaborative management,* ed 3, St Louis, 1995, Mosby.

phoresis, and hemorrhage. Hypovolemia is primarily treated with crystalloids, although colloids such as albumin may be added. A large volume of parenteral fluids will be required if shock is present. No oral fluids are administered until the patient is pain free and has bowel sounds. Calcium, potassium, and magnesium are added to intravenous (IV) fluids as needed (see Chapter 6).

2. **Hyponatremia** may develop because of loss of sodium-containing fluids, accompanied by hypovolemia-induced increase in antidiuretic hormone secretion (see Chapter 7).

3. **Hypocalcemia** caused by calcium deposition in areas of fat necrosis, decreased secretion of parathyroid hormone (PTH) (remember that PTH is the primary regulator of serum calcium levels), hypoalbuminemia, and ARF (if it develops). IV calcium gluconate is indicated for the treatment of significant or symptomatic hypocalcemia (see Chapter 9).

4. **Hypomagnesemia** caused by abnormal gastrointestinal (GI) losses and deposition of magnesium in areas of fat necrosis (see Chapter 11).

5. **Hypokalemia** may occur because of abnormal GI losses (see Chapter 8).

6. **Respiratory alkalosis** may develop in the patient with respiratory complications because of hypoxemia-induced hyperventilation (see Chapter 14).

7. **Parenteral feeding** is indicated for patients with severe pancreatitis (see Chapter 26).

# Hepatic Failure

24

Hepatic failure is a severe loss of liver function that may develop rapidly, as with viral or drug-induced (see the box on p. 234) hepatitis, or slowly, as with Laennec's cirrhosis. In the pediatric population, it may also occur as the result of Reye's syndrome or genetic disorders. As liver insufficiency progresses, normal functions of the liver, such as nutrient, hormone, and bilirubin metabolism, are lost. Elevated bilirubin levels, combined with decreased production of bile, lead to jaundice and a deficiency of the fat-soluble vitamins A, D, and K. Lack of adequate vitamin K, combined with decreased hepatic production of several clotting factors, decreased clearance of activated clotting factors, and thrombocytopenia, results in the bleeding tendency that is common in persons with hepatic failure. Decreased synthesis of albumin, in conjunction with intrahepatic vascular obstruction, contributes to the development of ascites and decreased intravascular volume (see discussion on p. 234). Reduced vascular volume stimulates the release of renin, angiotensin, aldosterone, and antidiuretic hormone (ADH), which collectively act on the kidneys to conserve sodium and water, potentiating the development of ascites and contributing to peripheral edema.

Loss of liver function results in dysfunction in other organs such as the brain, lungs, and kidneys. The damaged liver is unable to metabolize substances such as ammonia, which are toxic to the brain. Although the exact pathogenesis of hepatic encephalopathy remains unclear, elevated ammonia levels are associated with worsening encephalopathy. Hepatorenal syndrome, a type of acute renal failure that develops with advanced hepatic disease, is believed to develop because of unopposed renal vasoconstriction secondary to chronic release of renin, ADH, and norepinephrine. Decreased hepatic synthesis of prostaglandin precursors may limit normal renal protective mechanisms. Circulatory changes also occur in the lungs with the development of a significant ventilation-

## Drugs with Hepatotoxic Potential

| | |
|---|---|
| Acetaminophen | Methyldopa |
| Ampicillin | Monoamine oxidase |
| Carbamazepine | (MAO) inhibitors |
| Carbenicillin | Nonsteroidal antiinflam- |
| Carbon tetrachloride | matory drugs |
| Chloramphenicol | (NSAIDs) |
| Chlorpromazine | Oral contraceptives |
| Clindamycin | Penicillin |
| Cocaine | Phenytoin |
| Dantrolene | Propylthiouracil |
| Ethanol | Rifampin |
| FUDR (intraarterial) | Salicylates |
| Halothane | Sulfonamides |
| Hydrochlorothiazide | Tetracyclines (espe- |
| Isoniazid | cially parenteral) |
| Ketoconazole | Valproic acid |
| Methotrexate | |

From Keen JH: Gastrointestinal dysfunctions. In Swearingen PL, Keen JH, editors: *Manual of critical care nursing: nursing interventions and collaborative management,* ed 3, St Louis, 1995, Mosby.

perfusion mismatch. Hyperventilation and respiratory alkalosis are also common.

## Potential Fluid, Electrolyte, and Acid-Base Disturbances

1. **Alterations in fluid volume** may be present as evidenced by ascites and peripheral edema. Ascites occurs in cirrhosis because of hepatic venous obstruction and retention of sodium and water by the kidney, which together increase the hydrostatic pressure in the sinusoids, favoring movement of fluid into the peritoneal space. The increased sodium and water retention that occurs with ascites is believed to be caused both by abnormal handling of sodium and water by the kidney (the overflow or overfill theory) and compensatory retention of sodium and water caused by a reduction in effective circulating volume (ECV) that stimulates the renin-aldosterone system (the underfill theory). Reduction in ECV is the result of decreased hepatic synthesis of albumin (remember that

albumin helps hold the vascular volume in the vascular space), peripheral vasodilation, and ascites formation itself. An increase in pressure within the peritoneal cavity caused by ascities results in increased femoral venous pressure. This, combined with hypoalbuminemia, leads to the development of peripheral edema. Edema may be treated with fluid and sodium restriction and potassium-sparing diuretics. Potassium-wasting diuretics usually are avoided because of the risk of hypokalemic metabolic alkalosis. Massive or tense ascites may require paracentesis. A peritoneovenous shunt, which drains ascitic fluid into the internal jugular vein, may be indicated for patients with refractory ascites complicated by hepatorenal syndrome. (See Chapter 6 for a discussion of hypervolemia, edema, and diuretics.) Note that intravascular hypovolemia may develop with excessive use of diuretics or rapid removal of ascitic fluid.

2. **Hyponatremia** is common in cirrhotic patients with ascites and edema, especially in the terminal stage. Hyponatremia is dilutional and is the result of abnormal renal handling of water (see Chapter 7).

3. **Hypokalemia** is commonly seen in the cirrhotic patient with ascites and edema. Causes of hypokalemia in these individuals include poor dietary intake, administration of potassium-wasting diuretics, elevated aldosterone levels (remember that aldosterone causes an increased urinary excretion of potassium), magnesium depletion (hypomagnesemia often is associated with hypokalemia), and vomiting. NOTE: Hypokalemia may cause an increase in serum ammonia levels and precipitate hepatic coma. Use of potassium-sparing diuretics helps prevent hypokalemia (see Chapter 8).

4. **Hyperkalemia** may occur when the liver disease is complicated by renal failure or inappropriate use of potassium-sparing diuretics (see Chapter 6 for a discussion of diuretic therapy and see Chapter 8).

5. **Hypocalcemia** may occur in alcoholic cirrhosis as the result of magnesium depletion (hypomagnesemia causes a reduction in the release and action of parathyroid hormone) or poor oral intake (see Chapter 10).

6. **Hypomagnesemia** may occur in alcoholic cirrhosis because of poor oral intake, decreased gastrointestinal (GI) absorption, abnormal GI losses, and increased urinary excretion (see Chapter 11).

7. **Hypophosphatemia** occurs with chronic alcoholism, especially during acute withdrawal, secondary to poor dietary intake, increased GI losses with vomiting and diarrhea, use of phosphorus-binding antacids, hyperventilation (respiratory alkalosis causes an intracellular shift of phosphorus), and increased urinary losses (see Chapter 10).

8. **Respiratory alkalosis** may occur in all types of liver disease as the result of direct stimulation of the medullary respiratory center. Alkalosis increases the cellular uptake of ammonia and, combined with hypokalemia, may precipitate hepatic coma (see Chapter 14).

9. **Metabolic alkalosis** also may occur in the setting of liver failure as a result of diuretic therapy (see Chapter 6 for a discussion of metabolic alkalosis and diuretic therapy and see Chapter 16).

10. **Metabolic acidosis** may develop in severe chronic liver disease because of the liver's inability to metabolize lactic acid, the presence of alcoholic-induced and starvation-induced ketoacidosis, renal failure with the retention of acids, and the loss of bicarbonate in diarrhea (see Chapter 15).

# Burns

**25**

The skin is a complex organ that provides the body's first line of defense against a potentially hostile environment. It protects against infection, prevents loss of body fluids, helps control body temperature, functions as an excretory and sensory organ, aids in activating vitamin D, and influences body image. Burns are a common, yet largely preventable form of skin injury. In the initial phase of thermal injury, marked shifts in fluids and electrolytes pose the greatest risk to recovery. The immediate goal of therapy for major burns is preservation of vital organ function in the presence of significant hypovolemia and acidosis. The challenge of treatment is to maintain vascular volume and tissue perfusion with a minimum of edema formation.

In burns covering less than 30% of the body, fluid shifts are limited to the area of burn injury. Injured tissues release chemical mediators that increase local capillary permeability, allowing both colloids and crystalloids to move into the interstitial space. Increased capillary permeability is greatest during the first 8 to 12 hours postburn, although full recovery of capillary integrity does not occur for 2 to 3 days. When burns cover more than 30% of the body, fluid shifts occur in both burned and nonburned tissue. The edema that develops in nonburned tissue is believed to be caused largely by hypoproteinemia resulting from loss of protein into burned tissue and to a lesser extent by the action of circulating vasoactive substances. In addition, thermal injury decreases cell membrane potential, allowing sodium and water to enter the cells, causing cellular swelling. The loss of skin also leads to a direct loss of fluid and heat from the body. Metabolic acidosis develops because of decreased tissue perfusion. Inhalation injury or injury to the upper airways with development of tissue edema limits the ability of the lungs to compensate for acidosis via hyperventilation. Severe inhalation injury may lead to profound hypoxemia and respiratory acidosis that require mechanical ventilation.

Table 25-1    Characteristics of burn wound depth

| Criterion | Partial Thickness | Full Thickness |
|---|---|---|
| Cause | Flash, flame, ultra-violet (sunburn), hot liquid or solid, chemicals, radiation | Extended contact with flame, hot liquid or solid, steam, chemical, electric, radiation |
| Surface appearance | *Superficial:* Dry, no blisters or edema *Deep:* Moist blebs, blisters, edema, oozing of plasma-like fluid | Dry, leathery, eschar; thrombosed blood vessels may be visible |
| Color | Cherry red to mottled white; will blanch and refill | Ranges in color from red to khaki; waxy; charred; does not blanch |
| Sensation | *Superficial:* Very painful to the touch *Deep:* Extremely sensitive to touch, temperature, and air currents | Anesthetized to touch and temperature because of destruction of sensory nerve endings |
| Healing | 3-35 days | Grafting required for wounds ≥4 cm |

From Johnson J: Burns. In Swearingen PL, Keen JH, editors: *Manual of critical care nursing: nursing interventions and collaborative management,* ed 3, St Louis, 1995, Mosby.

Burns are classified according to wound depth and are described either as partial-thickness or full-thickness burns, depending on the layer of skin involved. Partial-thickness burns, which involve the epidermis, may be either superficial (i.e., dry, without blisters and edema) or deep (i.e., moist, with blisters, blebs, and edema and involving the epidermis and varying levels of the dermis). Full-thickness burns destroy all epidermal elements and require skin grafting if they are larger than 4 cm in diameter (see Table 25-1 for characteristics of the various types of burns).

One of the first steps in burn therapy is to determine the extent of the burn wound (Figures 25-1 and 25-2) and magnitude of the burn injury (Table 25-2). Burn magnitude and severity determines

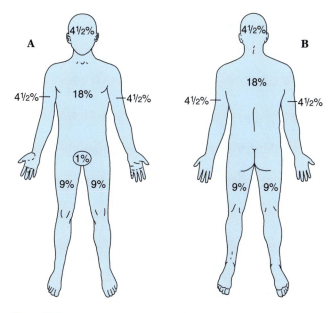

Figure 25-1
Estimation of adult burn injury: rule of nines. **A,** Anterior view. **B,** Posterior view.

whether the patient requires transfer to a specialized burn center for treatment (see the box on p. 242 for factors that determine burn severity). Knowledge of the extent of the burn wound is essential in estimating the volume of fluid needed to replace that which is lost into the tissues.

Aggressive fluid replacement is necessary during the initial resuscitation phase. Several formulas advocating the use of both crystalloids and colloids have been developed to direct fluid therapy (Table 25-3). Some formulas recommend crystalloids for the first 24 hours with a switch primarily to colloids on the second day. Others recommend the use of both crystalloids and colloids during the first 24 hours postburn. In either case, the key to effective treatment is the tailoring of fluid therapy to the individual's need and response to fluid replacement.

Mobilization of edema begins at approximately 72 hours postburn. Intravascular fluid overload with congestive heart failure

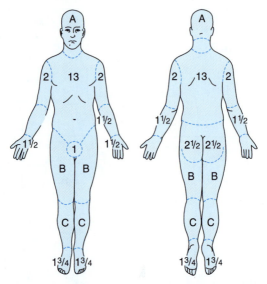

Relative percentages of areas affected by growth
(age in years)

|  | 0 | 1 | 5 | 10 | 15 | Adult |
|---|---|---|---|---|---|---|
| Half of head | 9½ | 8½ | 6½ | 5½ | 4½ | 3½ |
| Half of thigh | 2¾ | 3¼ | 4 | 4¼ | 4½ | 4¾ |
| Half of leg | 2½ | 2½ | 2¾ | 3 | 3¼ | 3½ |

Second degree _____ and
Third degree   _____ =
Total percent burned _____

Figure 25-2
Estimation of burn injury: Lund and Browder chart. Areas
designated by letters (*A, B,* and *C*) represent percentages of
body surface area that vary according to age. Accompanying table indicates relative percentages of these areas at various stages in life.

is a risk at this time. Because the body must rid itself of excess fluid
that was required during the initial acute phase, massive diuresis of
fluid is expected, and this loss should not be replaced fully. Careful
monitoring of hemodynamic status is essential during this phase to
prevent dangerous fluid volume changes.

**Table 25-2** American Burn Association classification system

| Magnitude of Burn Injury | Partial Thickness | | Full Thickness Adults and Children (% BSA) | Special Location* | Complications, Poor Risk, Fractures, Other Trauma |
|---|---|---|---|---|---|
| | Adult (% BSA) | Children (% BSA) | | | |
| Major | >25% | >20% | >10% | + | + |
| Moderate | 15%-25% | 10%-20% | 2%-10% | − | − |
| Minor | <15% | <10% | <2% | − | − |

From Johnson J: Burns. In Swearingen PL, Keen JH, editors: *Manual of critical care nursing: nursing interventions and collaborative management*, ed 3, St Louis, 1995, Mosby.

*Special location: Hands, face, eyes, feet, and/or genitalia.

*BSA*, Body surface area.

## Factors Determining Burn Severity

| | |
|---|---|
| Extent | Severity dependent on intensity and duration of exposure |
| Depth | Severity dependent on intensity and duration of exposure |
| Age | Patients <2 years old and >60 years old |
| Medical history | Preexisting conditions such as heart disease and chronic renal failure |
| Body part | Special burn areas: hands, face, eyes, ears, feet, and genitalia |
| Complications | Burns with concomitant trauma (i.e., fractures) |

From Johnson J: Burns. In Swearingen PL, Keen JH, editors: *Manual of critical care nursing: nursing interventions and collaborative management,* ed 3, St Louis, 1995, Mosby.

# Potential Fluid, Electrolyte, and Acid-Base Disturbances

1. **Hypovolemia** caused by increased capillary permeability, with loss of intravascular fluid and proteins into the interstitium, and evaporative loss of fluid through the burn wound. The plasma-to-interstitial fluid shift occurs during the first 2 to 3 days. Later, there is a shift of fluid from the interstitium back into the plasma. **Hypervolemia** may develop at this time, especially if there has been aggressive fluid replacement during the initial phase. As discussed, fluid replacement may involve the use of both crystalloids (usually lactated Ringer's solution) and colloids (usually albumin). Hypertonic sodium chloride solutions have been advocated by some burn centers (see Chapter 6).

2. **Hyponatremia** caused by hypovolemia-induced increase in antidiuretic hormone (ADH). Sodium chloride is administered to maintain the serum sodium level within an acceptable range (see Chapter 7).

3. **Hyperkalemia** caused by release of potassium from damaged cells. This is most likely to occur when the burn injury is complicated by acute renal failure. **Hypokalemia** may develop during the recovery phase because of shift of potassium back into the cells and increased excretion of potassium in the urine (see Chapter 8).

**Table 25-3** Formulas used in estimating fluid requirements for adults during the acute phase of burn injury

| Formula | First 24 hr | | | Second 24 hr | | |
|---|---|---|---|---|---|---|
| | Crystalloid/Electrolyte Solution | Colloid-Containing Fluid/Plasma Equivalent | Dextrose in Water | Crystalloid/Electrolyte Solution | Colloid-Containing Fluid/Plasma Equivalent | Dextrose in Water |
| Parkland | Lactated Ringer's 4 ml/kg/% TBSA burned | | | | 20%-60% of calculated plasma volume | As necessary for maintaining urinary output |
| Brooke | Lactated Ringer's 1.5 ml/kg/% TBSA burned | 0.5 ml/kg/% TBSA burned | 2 L | ½-¾ of first 24-hr requirement | ½-¾ of first 24-hr requirement | 2 L |
| Modified Brooke | Lactated Ringer's 2 ml/kg/% TBSA burned | | | | 0.3-0.5 ml/kg/% TBSA burn | As necessary for maintaining urinary output |
| Evans | Normal saline 1 ml/kg/% TBSA burned | 1 ml/kg/% TBSA burned; dextran 70 in normal saline or whole blood | 2 L | ½ of first 24-hr requirement | ½ of first 24-hr requirement | 2 L |

From Johnson J: Burns. In Swearingen PL, Keen JH, editors: *Manual of critical care nursing: nursing interventions and collaborative management*, ed 3, St Louis, 1995, Mosby.

*TBSA*, Total body surface area.

4. **Hypocalcemia** may develop because of loss of extracellular fluid from the burn wound and shift of calcium to the wound (see Chapter 9).

5. **Hypophosphatemia** commonly is associated with burns and occurs several days after the burn injury. The exact cause is unknown, but it may occur because of elevated calcitonin levels or respiratory alkalosis (see Chapter 10).

6. **Metabolic acidosis** may occur because of the release of acids from damaged tissue and production of lactic acid if hypovolemia has led to shock. Metabolic acidosis can be avoided or minimized by early treatment of fluid volume deficit (see Chapter 15).

7. **Respiratory alkalosis** may develop because of hyperventilation secondary to pain and anxiety (see Chapter 14).

8. **Respiratory acidosis** may develop with severe inhalation injury (see Chapter 13).

# Providing Nutritional Support

## 26

The body adapts to altered nutritional status through a series of changes to compensate for the decreased intake and absorption or increased excretion of important nutrients. In patients with a fluid and electrolyte disturbance, the nurses' role is not only to assist with identification and implementation of interventions for at-risk patients but also to continually evaluate the effectiveness of the prescribed interventions to resolve both the electrolyte and nutritional disturbance.

## Nutritional Assessment

Sources of information include any and all of the following: historic data, nutritional history, anthropometric data, biochemical analysis of blood and urine, and duration of the disease process.

### Nutritional History

In a nutritional history, the adequacy of usual and recent food intake is investigated and anything that has impaired adequate selection, preparation, ingestion, digestion, absorption, and excretion of nutrients before admission is noted. If possible, a 3-day calorie count in patients who can eat should be carried out. The patient should be asked about the following:

- The patient's usual dietary intake, noting food allergies, food aversions, and the use of nutritional supplements
- Recent unplanned weight gain or loss
- Chewing or swallowing difficulties
- Nausea, vomiting, or pain with eating
- Alteration in elimination pattern (e.g., constipation or diarrhea)
- Chronic disease affecting use of nutrients (e.g., malabsorption,

pancreatitis, diabetes mellitus, chronic renal failure)
- Recent trauma, operation, or period of sepsis
- Use of medications (e.g., analgesics, antacids, antibiotics, antineoplastic drugs), laxatives, and alcohol

Excesses or deficiencies of nutrients and any special eating patterns (various types of vegetarian or prescribed diets), use of fad diets, or excessive supplementation should be noted.

## Physical Assessment

Most physical findings are not conclusive for particular nutritional deficiencies. In particular, the following should be noted:
- Loss of muscle and adipose tissue (weight changes)
- Work and muscle endurance (easily fatigued)
- Changes in hair (easy pluckability), skin (poor wound healing), or neuromuscular function (weakness)

## Anthropometric Data

*Anthropometrics* is the measurement of the body or its parts. It is helpful to remember that 1 L of fluid equals approximately 2 lbs. Pounds and inches are converted to metric measurements using the following formulas:
- Divide pounds by 2.2 to convert to kilograms (kg)
- Divide inches by 39.37 to convert to meters (m)

## Height

Height is used to determine ideal weight and body mass index (BMI).
- Obtain an estimate from the family or significant others.
- Compare the patient's recumbent length with the known length of the mattress.

## Weight

Weight is a readily available and practical indicator of nutritional status and should be compared with previous weight or ideal weight or used to calculate BMI. Changes may reflect fluid retention (edema, third spacing), fluid depletion (diuresis, dehydration), surgical resections, traumatic amputations, or the weight of dressings or equipment. The actual body weight should be used to avoid overfeeding in starved patients, and ideal body weight should be used in patients who weigh more than 120% of their ideal body weight.

## Body Mass Index

BMI is used to evaluate adult weight. One calculation and one set of standards are applicable for both men and women.

$$\text{BMI (kg/m}^2) = \frac{\text{Weight (kg)}}{\text{Height (m)} \times \text{Height (m)}}$$

BMI values of 20 to 25 are optimum; values greater than 25 indicate obesity; and values less than 20 indicate underweight status.

## Triceps Skin Fold Thickness

- Calipers are used to measure the skin thickness over the triceps muscle of the nondominant upper arm halfway between the shoulder and the elbow.
- Because of the variation between clinicians, the position of the patient, the site of measurement, and the patient's age and fluid status, it is difficult to obtain accurate results.
- Accuracy can be increased when the same nurse, specially trained clinicians, or dietitians carry out the procedure (<3 mm indicates severely depleted fat stores).

## Biochemical Data

No laboratory test specifically measures nutritional status. Use the following to obtain an estimate:

### Protein status

1. **Albumin:** Has a relatively long half-life of 20 days, thus it is a less sensitive index of current nutritional status, although it remains a critical nutritional marker. Normal range is 3.5 to 5.5 g/dl.
2. **Transferrin:** With a half-life of 8 days, this globulin protein, to which iron is bound, is a powerful indicator (in the absence of anemia) of current nutritional status. In the presence of iron deficiency anemia, there is an increase in transferrin concentration, which decreases its sensitivity as a nutritional marker. Normal range is 250 to 420 mg/dl.
3. **Thyroxine-binding albumin:** With a half-life of 24 to 48 hours, it correlates closely with transferrin levels and nitrogen balance and is a sensitive marker of nutritional status. Its use may be affected by its cost and availability. Normal range is 10 to 40 mg/dl.

# Nitrogen balance studies

A positive nitrogen balance (the goal of nutritional therapy) is present when nitrogen intake is greater than its excretion, resulting in an anabolic state. If more nitrogen is excreted than is taken in, nitrogen balance is said to be negative, and a catabolic state exists. Most nitrogen loss occurs through the urine, with a small, constant amount lost via the skin and feces. Nitrogen balance studies should be performed by specialists as an accurate measurement of 24-hour food intake and urine output is required.

# Creatinine-height index

Comparison of a patient's 24-hour urinary creatinine excretion with a predicted urinary creatinine for persons with the same height evaluates body muscle mass. The quantity of creatinine produced is directly related to skeletal muscle wasting. The validity of results is affected by inaccuracies in the urine collection procedure and the lack of age-referenced norms. Normal range of 80% to 100% reflects adequate muscle mass.

# Estimating Nutritional Requirements

The primary goal of nutritional support is to meet the energy needs for body temperature, metabolic processes, and tissue repair. Energy needs can be estimated using the Harris and Benedict equation; indirect calorimetry; distribution of calories; special diets for organ-specific pathologic conditions; electrolytes, vitamins, and essential trace mineral requirements; and fluid requirements.

# Harris and Benedict equation

A commonly used method to determine basal energy expenditure (BEE) is calculated using the following equations developed by Harris and Benedict:

BEE (male) = $66.5 + (13.8 \times W) + (5 \times H) - (6.8 \times A)$

BEE (female) = $655.1 + (9.6 \times W) + (1.9 \times H) - (4.7 \times A)$

*W,* Weight in kg; *H,* height in cm; *A,* age in years.

The amount of required calories per day is expressed as BEE. Then BEE is multiplied by a stress factor that is estimated from the degree of stress and the need for weight maintenance or repletion. Multiplying the BEE by 1.2 to 1.5 provides a range appropriate for most patients. The lower factor is appropriate for patients without significant stress, whereas the higher factor is appropriate for patients with higher levels of stress such as trauma or sepsis. Patients with burns may require even higher stress factors (e.g., 2 to 3 times the caloric requirements of the BEE).

## Indirect calorimetry

Indirect calorimetry is a sophisticated specialized technique to measure energy needs using a bedside metabolic cart. Carts are an expense most units cannot justify.

## Distribution of calories

A relatively normal distribution of calories usually is adequate (e.g., carbohydrates, protein, and fat should equal approximately 55%, 15%, and 30%, respectively). To avoid overfeeding, 30 to 35 kcal/kg is appropriate for most critically ill patients.

1. **Protein requirements:** Usually are 1.5 to 2 g/kg/day.
2. **Carbohydrate requirements:** Glucose administration of 5 mg/kg/min is a suitable amount. Carbohydrates provided in excess are not well used and may lead to hyperglycemia, excessive carbon dioxide ($CO_2$) production, hypophosphatemia, and fluid overload.
3. **Fat requirements:** If protein and glucose are supplied as outlined, the remainder of needed calories can be supplied by fat. Fat can be administered in minimal quantities to satisfy needs for essential fatty acids, or it can be offered in larger quantities, as tolerated, to meet energy needs. Abnormal liver function often occurs in patients maintained on total parenteral nutrition (TPN) longer than 3 weeks. Usually the enzymes return to normal on cessation of TPN. Giving cyclic TPN, in which the patient receives TPN for 12 to 16 hours out of 24 hours, sometimes helps.

## Special diets for organ-specific pathologic conditions

Special diets for organ-specific pathologic conditions are costly, and the metabolic advantages of some products remain controversial.

1. **Hepatic failure:** For patients with hepatic encephalopathy (unresponsive to medical therapy with lactulose or neomycin), a product containing a liver-specific amino acid mixture should be used. General use for all patients with liver disease has not been shown to be more effective.

2. **Renal disease:** High percentages of essential amino acids are used for short periods to improve nitrogen use and to decrease urea formation. Patients with chronic renal failure with a superimposed acute illness may benefit from special mixtures.

3. **Respiratory disease:** A low-protein and low-carbohydrate diet may decrease $CO_2$ production and, consequently, the work of breathing in some patients.

## Electrolytes, vitamins, and essential trace mineral requirements

Potassium, calcium, magnesium and phosphorus may need to be provided to keep levels within the normal range. In general, follow the Recommended Daily Allowance (RDA) to provide minimum quantities of vitamins and trace minerals. For specific patients, specific vitamins or minerals needed may be supplemented in increased amounts for existing disease states (e.g., zinc and vitamins A and C for burns; thiamine, folate, and vitamin $B_{12}$ for chronic alcohol ingestion).

## Fluid requirements

Many factors affect fluid balance. All sources of intake (oral, enteral, intravenous, and medications), as well as output (urine, stool, drainage, emesis, fluid shifts, and respiratory and evaporate losses), must be considered.

# Nutritional Support Modalities

Cost, safety, and convenience have been the rationale for enteral nutrition over parenteral nutrition support, but the physiologic benefits are a more compelling argument. Studies indicate that enteral feeding prevents passage of bacteria from the gastrointestinal (GI) tract into the lymphatic system and other organs, reducing a major source of sepsis and possible organ failure, while fostering wound healing and immunocompetence.

## Enteral Nutrition

Enteral nutrition is that which is provided via the GI tract. Oral enteral nutrition is taken by mouth; tube enteral nutrition is provided through a tube or catheter that delivers nutrients distal to the oral cavity.

## Types of feeding tubes and sites

1. **Stomach:** Easiest for tube placement, simulates normal GI function, and may be used for intermittent or continuous feedings. The stomach is the site best reserved for patients who are alert, with intact gag and cough reflexes. Entry site is nasal, oral, or stomach.
   - *Small bore:* Soft polyurethane or silicone with or without tungsten tip; designed for long-term use; size 6Fr to 12Fr; length 20 to 45 inches. Trade names include Keofeed and ENtube. Some nasoenteric feeding tubes have a Y port, allowing irrigation and medication administration without disconnecting the administration set. Flexiflow is one example.
   - *Large bore:* Stiff polyvinyl chloride; size 10Fr to 18Fr; used for short-term feeding of highly viscous fluids. One trade name is Levine.
   - *Combination:* An inner soft silicone tube may be contained within a stiff outer tube that is removed, leaving the inner soft tube in place, or the tube may have a rigid guide wire that is removed after insertion. This tube is easier to place.
   - *Gastrostomy tube:* A soft tube, often a Foley catheter size 18Fr to 24Fr, is inserted directly into the stomach either temporarily or permanently.
   - *Percutaneous endoscopic gastrostomy (PEG) tubes:* A soft tube that is inserted into the stomach via the esophagus, then drawn through the abdominal skin using a stab incision.

2. **Small bowel:** Used for patients with diminished protective pharyngeal reflexes; the small bowel is less affected than the stomach and colon by postoperative ileus. Tube placement is more difficult. Continuous feedings are tolerated better as the continuous drip approximates normal function. Entry sites are nasal, oral, duodenum, and jejunum.
   - *Small bore:* See "Stomach," discussed previously. Some tubes have one port for feeding into the jejunum and a second port for aspiration and decompression of the stomach.
   - *Duodenum/jejunum:* Minimizes risk of vomiting and aspiration compared with gastric feedings. A jejunostomy tube is soft, is inserted into the jejunum, and is not easily dislodged. Needle catheter (Witzel) jejunostomy is an

alternative method of nutrient delivery and is often placed at the time of surgery.

## Infusion rates

Table 26-1 provides the methods and rates of administration of enteral products.

Table 26-1    Methods and rates of administration for enteral products

| Type | Description | Comments |
|------|-------------|----------|
| Bolus | 250-400 ml 4-6 ×/day | May cause cramping, bloating, dumping; not recommended |
| Intermittent | 120 ml isotonic formula with 30-50 ml $H_2O$ flush over 30-60 minutes | Starting regimen |
| | Advancement: Increase formula q8-12h by 60 ml if residual < half the volume of previous feeding | Should not exceed 30 ml/min; may cause cramping, nausea, bloating, diarrhea, aspiration; useful for ambulatory patients |
| Continuous | 40-50 ml/hr, full strength, isotonic formula | Starting regimen |
| | Advancement: Increase by 25 ml q8h; if serum albumin levels <2.5 g/dl or initial loose stools, dilute formula to ½ strength | Used for feeding into small intestine |

From Webber KS: Nutritional support. In Swearingen PL, Keen JH, editors: *Manual of critical care nursing: nursing interventions and collaborative management,* ed 3, St Louis, 1995, Mosby.

# Enteral products

Enteral products are composed of a wide variety of standard and modular formulas (Table 26-2).

## Formula types

1. **Standard:** Commercial formulas that are sterile, homogenous, suitable for small-bore feeding tubes, and have a fixed nutrient composition and blended whole food diets, which are less costly but have problems that include possible bacterial growth, solids that settle out, variation in nutrient composition, and the necessity of a large-bore tube for the viscous solution.
2. **Modular:** Consists of a single nutrient that may be combined with other modules (nutrients) to form a package designed for an individual's specific deficits (e.g., carbohydrate, fat protein, and vitamin modules).

## Nutritional composition

1. **Carbohydrate:** The most easily digested and absorbed component in enteral formulas; 80% of all carbohydrate is broken down and absorbed as simple glucose in the normal intestine.
2. **Lactase:** An enzyme that aids in the digestion of lactose. It is most commonly deficient in African Americans, Asians, Native Americans, and Jews. A secondary form may also be found in individuals for whom large amounts of lactose are given in a milk-based diet. Symptoms include watery diarrhea, abdominal cramps, flatulence, fullness, nausea, stool with a pH of less than 6, and stool that tests positive for glucose.
3. **Fiber:** Now included in many commercial preparations because it is claimed to be helpful in controlling blood glucose, reducing hyperlipidemia, and controlling diarrhea. These preparations are highly viscous and require a large-bore feeding tube such as a 10Fr or an infusion pump. Begin the infusion slowly to reduce transient symptoms of gas and abdominal distention.
4. **Protein:** Three forms are commonly used.
   - *Polymeric:* Protein found in complete and original form (e.g., commercial and blenderized whole food diets that require normal levels of pancreatic enzymes).

Table 26-2   Types of enteral formulations

| Enteral Formula | Description |
|---|---|
| **Blended Diets** | |
| Compleat (regular and modified), Vitaneed | Nutritionally complete, requiring complete digestive capabilities, composed of all natural food groups, including meat, vegetables, milk, and fruit |
| **Milk-based Formulas** | |
| Meritene, Sustagen, Carnation Instant (if mixed with milk) | Nutritionally adequate diet for general nutritional support |
| **Lactose-free Formulas** | |
| Ensure, Entrition 1 Isocal, Osmolite | Nutritionally adequate, liquid preparation, used for general nutritional support, isoosmolar or hypoosmolar, all except Osmolite are low residue |
| **Elemental or Chemically Defined Formulas** | |
| Criticare | Nutrients are tailored for specific needs (e.g., low-sodium, lactose-free, high-nitrogen diet), 40% of protein is supplied as small peptides, nutritionally adequate, used for general nutritional support |
| Travasorb HN | Nutritionally adequate, used for general nutritional support, containing additional hydrolyzed protein that is readily digested and rapidly absorbed |
| **Specialty Formulas** | |
| *Hepatic failure* | |
| Hepatic Travasorb | Nutritionally complete; contains a greater ratio of branched-chain to aromatic amino acids and restricts total amino acid concentrations, added nonprotein calories |

Table 26-2    Types of enteral formulations—cont'd

| Enteral Formula | Description |
|---|---|
| Hepatic-Aid II | Nutritionally incomplete powder formula with essential nutrient in easily digestible form; high in branched-chain amino acids; low in aromatic amino acids and methionine |
| *Renal failure* | |
| Renal Travasorb | Contains no electrolytes, lactose, or fat-soluble vitamins; high in calories; contains mostly essential amino acids; restricted total protein content may reduce or postpone the need for dialysis |
| Amin-Aid | Nutritionally incomplete powder supplement with essential nutrients and minimal electrolytes in readily digestible form |
| *Respiratory insufficiency* | |
| Pulmocare | Nutritionally complete, contains a higher proportion of fat-to-carbohydrate ratio to reduce $CO_2$ production |
| Modular Formulas | Offers highly flexible tailoring of nutrients (e.g., fat [Lipomul], protein [Pro Mod], and carbohydrate [Moducal] for specific needs) |

- *Hydrolyzed:* Protein that is broken down into smaller forms to assist absorption. It is helpful for short bowel syndrome or pancreatic insufficiency.
- *Elemental:* Protein that requires no further digestion and is ready for absorption. It is most useful in hepatic and renal disorders.
  5. **Fat:** Two forms are the primary sources.
- *Long-chain triglycerides (LCT):* A major source of essential fatty acids, fat soluble vitamins, and calories but is less easily absorbed.
- *Medium-chain triglycerides (MCT):* Foster the absorption of fat better than LCT but have side effects of nausea and vomiting, abdominal distention, and diarrhea.

## Managing complications

See Table 26-3.

## Parenteral Nutrition

Parenteral nutrition is the provision of some or all nutrients by central venous catheter (CVC) or peripheral venous catheter (PVC) to meet total nutritional needs in patients who cannot be given enteral support or to supplement patients who cannot absorb enough calories using the GI tract. Parenteral nutrition is more expensive and has more serious complications than enteral nutrition.

### Selection of feeding site

1. **CVC:** Used for infusion of large amounts of nutrients or electrolytes with smaller fluid volumes (hypertonic solutions) than with peripheral parenteral nutrition. The solution usually is delivered through a large-diameter vein (e.g., superior vena cava via the subclavian or jugular vein). The volume of blood flow rapidly dilutes the hypertonic solutions and decreases the irritation of vein walls. However, there are more complications than with the peripheral route.

2. **PVC:** The need for low osmolality of solutions (<800 mOsm/L) can limit usefulness. However, combining solutions of dextrose, amino acids, and lipids lowers the osmolality, providing a concentrated energy source that can be delivered through a peripheral vein, usually of the hand or forearm. This method is usually reserved for individuals who need partial or total nutritional support for short periods and for whom CVC access is unavailable.

### Types of catheters

See Table 26-4.

### Monitoring infusion rates

Using an infusion pump, parenteral nutrition is given at a consistent rate, with gradual acceleration on initiation or deceleration on cessation over a 3-day period to avoid wide fluctuations in blood glucose. A typical rate is 50 to 100 ml/hr, which increases 25 to 50 ml/hr/day depending on the patient's status.

## Table 26-3 Management of complications in the tube-fed patient

| Possible Causes | Suggested Management Strategy |
| --- | --- |
| Gastrointestinal/Pulmonary Complications | |
| *Nausea and vomiting* | |
| Fast rate | Decrease rate |
| Fat intolerance | Decrease fat proportion to 30% of total intake |
| Lactose intolerance | As prescribed, change to lactose-free product |
| Hyperosmolality | Dilute feeding |
| Delayed gastric emptying | Feed beyond the pylorus via naso-duodenal or jejunostomy tube; give metoclopramide to treat or prevent decreased peristalsis as prescribed |
| Product odor | Mask with flavoring |
| *Diarrhea* | |
| Lactose intolerance | Switch to lactose-free products as prescribed |
| Fat intolerance | Reduce fat intake during acute illness |
| Osmolality intolerance | Dilute feeding or use product with lower osmolality as prescribed |
| Low fiber content | Try bulk-forming agents (e.g., Metamucil) or switch to formula with added fiber |
| Medications | Review all medications patient is receiving; monitor use of sorbitol in liquid medications; dilute hypertonic oral liquids before administering; administer Lacto-bacillus acidophilus to restore GI flora as prescribed |

From Webber KS: Nutritional support. In Swearingen PL, Keen JH, editors: *Manual of critical care nursing: nursing interventions and collaborative management,* ed 3, St Louis, 1995, Mosby.

*Continued*

Table 26-3   Management of complications in the tube-fed patient—cont'd

| Possible Causes | Suggested Management Strategy |
|---|---|
| Bacterial contamination | Use full-strength, ready-to-use formula; discard feedings hanging for >8 hr (check manufacturers instructions for prefilled sets); wash hands well before handling equipment; wash intermittent delivery sets with hot soapy water and rinse after use, change equipment q24h, refrigerate all opened products but discard after 24 hr; administer medications via separate port |
| Low serum albumin | Low serum albumin levels contribute to intestinal malabsorption, monitor serum albumin level |
| *High gastric residual* | |
| Decreased motility | Hold feeding for 1 hr, and check residual repeat q1-2h until feedings can be resumed; have patient lie in right lateral position after feeding (head of bed 30 degrees), as prescribed; give metoclopramide |
| *Aspiration* | |
| Head of bed low | Raise head of bed 30 degrees during feeding and for 45 to 60 minutes after feeding, monitor breath sounds and vital signs. Test pulmonary secretions for glucose, which reflects the presence of formula (may be falsely positive when blood is in respiratory secretions). Monitor for the following signs: fever, unexplained pulmonary infiltrates, and increased respiratory rate and effort because aspiration can occur silently and quickly |
| Deflated endotracheal/ tracheostomy cuff | Keep cuff inflated during feeding |

**Table 26-3   Management of complications in the tube-fed patient—cont'd**

| Possible Causes | Suggested Management Strategy |
| --- | --- |
| Delayed gastric emptying | Feed beyond the pylorus via naso-duodenal or jejunostomy tube. As prescribed, give metoclopramide to treat or prevent decreased peristalsis |
| Incorrect tube position | Verify small-bore feeding tube position with x-ray scan. Auscultation of air into stomach is not the recommended procedure for placement verification. Aspiration of a small-bore tube causes collapse. Feed patients at risk for aspiration via small intestine |

Mechanical Complications

*Blocked tube*

| | |
| --- | --- |
| Viscous formula/ medications; inadequate flushing | Flush tube with 30 ml water before and after each checking of residuals; q4h during feeding; after medications |
| | Do not instill crushed medications in small-bore tubes. Substitute liquid preparations after consulting a pharmacist and the attending physician or crush into a very fine powder. Incompatibilities between drugs and feeding formulas are possible. Colas and cranberry juice have been suggested, but studies have not documented their superiority over water for flushing. Some studies suggest clearing blocked tubes with a meat tenderizer or a pancreatic enzyme; however, these practices are not fully evaluated. A device called Intro-Reducer has been designed to clear blocked soft feeding tubes, but efficacy is not documented |

Table 26-4    Catheters used in parenteral nutrition

| Catheter | Description |
|---|---|
| **Subclavian/Jugular** | |
| Single lumen | Soft, flexible, silicone catheter; considered less irritating and less thrombocytic, but kinks easily. Some catheters have a microbial cuff that provides a physical and chemical barrier to bacterial migration. Multiple uses for specimen retrieval, feeding, and medications administration increase the risk of infection, especially in compromised patients |
| Multilumen | Dedication of one lumen in a multilumen catheter is common practice, enabling other lumen(s) to be used for medication administration and laboratory monitoring |
| Right atrial catheter (e.g., Hickman, Broviac) | Composed of silicone rubber with plastic external segment; for long-term use |
| Implantable (e.g., Infuse-a-port, Port-a-Cath) | Designed for repeated access, making repeated venipuncture unnecessary |
| **Peripheral Devices** | |
| Dual lumen | Short-term use; allows dedication of one lumen for nutritional support and reserves second lumen for incompatible medications |

Modified from Webber KS: Providing nutritional support. In Swearingen PL, editor: *Manual of medical-surgical nursing care,* ed 3, St Louis, 1994, Mosby.

## Parenteral solutions

Parenteral solutions are derived from combinations of dextrose, amino acids, fat, electrolytes, vitamins, and trace elements. Total nutrient admixtures (TNAs) are formulated either by combining dextrose, fat, and amino acids in one container or, alternately, by combining dextrose and amino acid with a separate delivery device for fat. An in-line filter cannot be used with TNA because it would trap lipid molecules.

1. **Carbohydrate:** Dextrose solutions of 5% to 50% are used to meet part of the patient's energy needs. When hypertonic solutions are infused, insulin demand and $CO_2$ production and oxygen ($O_2$) consumption are increased, which may lead to respiratory distress and hypermetabolism.

2. **Protein:** Synthetic crystalline essential and nonessential amino acid formulations are available in concentrations of 3% to 15%. Special amino acid formulations for specific disorders are available (see p. 249).

3. **Fat:** Ten percent to twenty percent lipid is an isotonic solution providing essential fatty acids and a source of concentrated calories. For best use and tolerance, lipids should be infused with carbohydrates and protein over no less than 8 hours. The most common symptoms of an adverse reaction include febrile response, chills, shivering, and pain in the chest or back. A second type of adverse reaction occurs with prolonged use of intravenous fat emulsions and may result in a transient increase in liver enzymes, kernicterus, eosinophilia, and thrombophlebitis. Keep the infusion rate at 1 ml/min for the first 15 to 30 minutes and then increase to 80 to 100 ml/hr for the remainder of the first infusion.

## Managing complications

See Table 26-5.

# Transitional Feeding

A period of adjustment is needed before discontinuing nutrition support. Nutritional supplements should be tapered as oral intake increases. Patients receiving parenteral nutrition may have some mucosal atrophy of the bowel and may need a period of adjustment before the bowel can fully resume its usual functions of digestion and absorption.

## Potential Fluid, Electrolyte, and Acid-Base Disturbances
## Fluid Imbalances

1. **Hypervolemia:** Refeeding a malnourished individual results in raised insulin levels that decrease excretion of sodium by

Table 26-5   Management of complications in patients receiving parenteral nutrition

| Potential Complications | Management Strategy |
| --- | --- |
| Pneumothorax | Ensure that x-ray scan is done immediately after insertion. Determine placement of catheter before initiating feeding by observing for diminished or unequal breath sounds, tachypnea, dyspnea, and labored breathing. |
| Subclavian artery injury | If pulsatile, bright red blood returns into the syringe, assist physician with immediate removal of the needle and apply pressure for 10 minutes anteriorly and posteriorly at the point of penetration. |
| Catheter occlusion | If solution is infusing sluggishly, flush the line with heparinized saline. Check to see if line is kinked. If the line is occluded, try to aspirate clot and contact physician who may prescribe a thrombolytic agent. |
| Air embolism | Use Trendelenburg position when catheter is inserted into central vein. Have patient perform Valsalva's maneuver during tubing changes. Use Luer-Lok connections only to prevent disconnection; use occlusive dressing over insertion site for 24 hr after catheter has been removed to prevent air entry via catheter-sinus tract. If air embolism is suspected, place patient in left side-lying Trendelenburg position to trap air in the right ventricle; give oxygen and contact physician immediately. |

From Webber KS: Nutritional support. In Swearingen PL, Keen JH, editors: *Manual of critical care nursing: nursing interventions and collaborative management,* ed 3, St Louis, 1995, Mosby.

Table 26-5    Management of complications in patients receiving parenteral nutrition—cont'd

| Potential Complications | Management Strategy |
|---|---|
| Sepsis | Change catheter, catheter dressing, tubing, and filter according to agency policy. Tubing is usually changed every 2 days. Maintain strict aseptic technique with each dressing change, done usually every other day or as needed. |
| Hypoglycemia/ hyperglycemia | Administer 10% glucose solution in a peripheral vein if catheter becomes plugged or must be discontinued. Rapid increases or decreases are to be avoided. During early stages, monitor refeeding of malnourished patients carefully for high glucose levels. Monitor blood glucose via finger stick q6h or as needed until stable. |

the kidney. The retention of sodium and water is called *refeeding edema* (see Chapter 6).

2. **Hypovolemia:** Can occur in patients receiving increased amounts of protein in tube feeding and limited amounts of water. Also part of the refeeding syndrome (see Chapter 6).

## Electrolyte Imbalances

1. **Hypernatremia:** Refeeding stimulates movement of sodium ions from within the cell to the extracellular environment, increasing the levels of sodium; monitor all patients carefully for sodium intake from medications, blood products, and feedings (see Chapter 7).

2. **Hyponatremia:** Stable patients on long-term enteral feeding that contains limited sodium may experience hyponatremia (see Chapter 7).

3. **Hyperkalemia:** May be caused by excessive enteral or parenteral potassium supplementation. Hyperkalemia most often occurs in patients with metabolic acidosis and renal insufficiency (see Chapter 8).

4. **Hypokalemia:** Refeeding patients with marasmus may result in elevated plasma insulin that facilitates movement of potassium ions from the ECF into the cell, causing hypokalemia if replacement is insufficient (see Chapter 8).

5. **Hyperphosphatemia:** In tube-fed patients, hyperphosphatemia usually occurs as a result of renal dysfunction (see Chapter 10).

6. **Hypophosphatemia:** Occurs as a result of a complex process during refeeding a malnourished patient; the increased glucose levels elevate insulin levels, facilitating movement of phosphorus into intracellular space. Hypophosphatemia is accompanied by high mortality rate (see Chapter 10).

7. **Hypermagnesemia:** Transient elevations can occur with use of diuretics or extracellular volume depletion (see Chapter 11).

8. **Hypomagnesemia:** Also occurs as part of the refeeding syndrome. Insulin may increase uptake of magnesium in muscle cells, causing hypomagnesemia (see Chapter 11).

## Acid-Base Imbalance

**Respiratory acidosis:** May occur when high-carbohydrate enteral or parenteral nutrition is used secondary to increased $CO_2$ production.

# Selected References

Abraham WT, Schrier PW: Body fluid volume regulation in health and disease, *Adv Interm Med* 39:23-47, 1994.

Adrogué H, Wesson D: *Acid-base,* Boston, 1995, Blackwell Scientific Publications.

Altura BM, Altura BT: Cardiovascular risk factors and magnesium: relationships to atherosclerosis, ischemic heart disease and hypertension, *Magnes Trace Elem* 10:182-192, 1991-1992.

Arieff A: Acid-base, electrolyte, and metabolic abnormalities. In Parrillo J, Bone R, editors: *Critical care medicine: principles of diagnoses & management,* St Louis, 1995, Mosby.

Arieff A, Ayus JC: Pathogenesis of hyponatremic encephalopathy—current concepts, *Chest* 103(2):607-610, 1993.

Arsenian MA: Magnesium and cardiovascular disease, *Prog Cardiovasc Dis* 35(4):271-310, 1993.

ASPEN Board of Directors: Guidelines for the use of parenteral and enteral nutrition in adult and pediatric patients, *J Parenter Enteral Nutr* 17(4):1SA-25SA, 1993.

Baas L, Steuble BT: Cardiovascular dysfunctions. In Swearingen PL, Keen JH, editors: *Manual of critical care nursing: nursing interventions and collaborative management,* ed 3, St Louis, 1995, Mosby.

Bilezikian JP: Management of hypercalcemia, *J Clin Endocrinol Metab* 77(6):1445-1449, 1993.

Birney MH, Penney DG: Atrial natriuretic peptide: a hormone with implications for clinical practice, *Heart Lung* 19(2):174-185, 1990.

Bove LA: How fluids and electrolytes shift, *Nursing 94* 24(8):34-40, 1994.

Bourke E, Delaney V: Assessment of hypocalcemia and hypercalcemia, *Clin Lab Med* 13(1):157-181, 1993.

Bourke E, Yanagawa N: Assessment of hyperphosphatemia and hypophosphatemia, *Clin Lab Med* 13(1):183-207, 1993.

Brenner M, Wellever J: Pulmonary and acid-base assessment, *Nurs Clin North Am* 25(4):761-770, 1990.

Brown RG: Disorders of sodium balance, *Postgrad Med* 93(4):227-246, 1993.

Byers JF, Goshorn J: How to manage diuretic therapy, *Am J Nurs* 95(2):38-43, 1995.

Cogan MG: *Fluid and electrolytes—physiology and pathophysiology,* Norwalk, Conn and Los Altos, Calif, 1991, Appleton & Lange.

Corbett JV: *Laboratory tests and diagnostic procedures with nursing diagnoses,* ed 3, Norwalk, Conn and Los Altos, Calif, 1992, Appleton & Lange.

Dwyer K, Barone JE, Rogers JF: Severe hypophosphatemia in postoperative patients, *Nutr Clin Pract* 7:279-283, 1992.

Edes TE, Walk BE, Austin JL: Diarrhea in tube-fed patients: feeding formula not necessarily the cause, *Am J Med* 88(2):91-93, 1990.

Elin RJ: Magnesium: the fifth but forgotten electrolyte, *Am J Clin Pathol* 102(5):616-622, 1994.

Ewald GA, McKenzie CR, editors: *Manual of medical therapeutics,* ed 28, Boston, 1995, Little, Brown.

Feeney-Stewat F: The sodium bicarbonate controversy, *Dimen Crit Care* 9(1):22-27, 1990.

Gianino S, St. John RE: Nutritional assessment of the patient in the intensive care unit, *Crit Care Nurs Clin North Am* 5(1):1-16, 1993.

Goepp JG, Katz SA: Oral rehydration therapy, *Am Fam Physician* 47(4):843-848, 1994.

Guerci A: In CPR, look beyond bicarbonate, *Emerg Med* 24(7):223-225, 1995.

Hall TG, Schaiff RA: Update on the medical treatment of hypercalcemia of malignancy, *Clin Pharmacol Ther* 12:117-125, 1993.

Halperin MC, Goldstein MB: *Fluid, electrolyte, and acid-base physiology: a problem-based approach,* ed 2, Philadelphia, 1994, WB Saunders.

Handerhan B: Computing the anion gap, *RN* 54(7):30-31, 1991.

Hanson-Young M, Whitaker K: High output effluent management, *Ostomy/Wound Management* 29:30-38, 1990.

Heitz UE: Acid-base imbalances. In Swearingen PL, Keen JH, editors: *Manual of critical care nursing: nursing interventions and collaborative management,* ed 3, St Louis, 1995, Mosby.

Hodgson SF, Hurley DL: Acquired hypophosphatemia, *Endocrinol Metab Clin North Am* 22(2):397-409, 1993.

Holmes O: *Human acid-base physiology,* London, 1993, Chapman and Hall.

Horne MM: Endocrinologic dysfunctions. In Swearingen PL, Keen JH, editors: *Manual of critical care nursing: nursing interventions and collaborative management,* ed 3, St Louis, 1995, Mosby.

Horne MM: Fluid and electrolyte disturbances. In Swearingen PL, Keen JH, editors: *Manual of critical care nursing: nursing interventions and collaborative management,* ed 3, St Louis, 1995, Mosby.

Horne MM, Heitz UE, Swearingen PL: *Fluid, electrolyte, and acid-base balance—a case study approach,* St Louis, 1991, Mosby.

Hudak C, Gallo B: Critical care, ed 6, *Nursing: a holistic approach,* Philadelphia, 1994, JB Lippincott.

Ichikawa L: *Pediatric textbook of fluids and electrolytes,* Baltimore, 1990, Williams & Wilkins.

Imm A, Carlson RW: Fluid resuscitation in circulatory shock, *Crit Care Clin* 9(2):313-333, 1993.

Innerarity SA: Hyperkalemic emergencies, *Crit Care Nurs Q* 14(4):32-39, 1992.

Isselbache K et al, editors: *Harrison's principles of internal medicine,* ed 13, New York, 1994, McGraw-Hill Book.

Janusek L: Metabolic alkalosis, *Nursing 90* 20(6):52-53, 1990.

Jeejeebhoy KN, Detsky AS, Baker JP: Assessment of nutritional status, *J Parenter Enteral Nutr* 14(5):193S-196S, 1990.

Johnson J: Burns. In Swearingen PL, Keen JH, editors: *Manual of critical care nursing: nursing interventions and collaborative management,* ed 3, St Louis, 1995, Mosby.

Kaplan M: Hypercalcemia of malignancy: a review of advances in pathophysiology, *Oncol Nurs Forum* 21(6):1039-1046, 1994.

Keen JH: Gastrointestinal dysfunctions. In Swearingen PL, Keen JH, editors: *Manual of critical care nursing: nursing interventions and collaborative management,* ed 3, St Louis, 1995, Mosby.

Keithley JK, Eisenberg P: The significance of enteral nutrition in the intensive care unit patient, *Crit Care Nurs Clin North Am* 5(1):23-29, 1993.

Kim MJ, McFarland GK, McLane AM: *Pocket guide to nursing diagnoses,* ed 6, St Louis, 1995, Mosby.

Kitabchi AE, Wall BM: Diabetic ketoacidosis, *Med Clin North Am* 79(1):9-37, 1995.

Konstantinides NN, Lehmann S: The impact of nutrition on wound healing, *Crit Care Nurs* 13(5):25-33, 1993.

Kositzke JA: A question of balance—dehydration in the elderly, *J Gerontol* 16(5):4-11, 1990.

Kupin WL, Narvins RG: The hyperkalemia of renal failure: pathophysiology, diagnosis and therapy, *Contrib Nephrol* 102:1-22, 1993.

Lacey JA: Albumin overview: use as a nutritional marker and as a therapeutic intervention, *Crit Care Nurse* 11(1):46-49, 1991.

Levinsky NG: Acidoses and alkalosis. In Isselbache K et al, editors: *Harrison's principles of internal medicine,* ed 13, New York, 1994, McGraw-Hill Book.

Ljutic D, Rumboldt Z: Should glucose be administered before, with or after insulin, in the management of hyperkalemia? *Ren Fail* 15(1):73-76, 1993.

Lorber D: Nonketotic hyperosmolality in diabetes mellitus, *Med Clin North Am* 79(1):39-53, 1995.

Lovenstein J: *Acid and basics: a guide to understanding acid-based disorders,* New York, 1993, Oxford University.

Ludlow M: Renal handling of potassium, *ANNA J* 20(1): 52-56, 1993.

Manon SM, Casperson DS: Pathophysiology of hypokalemia in patients with cancer: implications for nurses, *MAHON* 20(6):937-946, 1993.

Marcuard SP, Stegall KS: Unclogging feeding tubes with pancreatic enzyme, *J Parenter Enteral Nutr* 14(2):198-200, 1990.

Marcuard SP, Stegall KS, Trogdon S: Clearing of obstructed feeding tubes, *J Parenter Enteral Nutr* 13(1):81-83, 1989.

Marik PE et al: Acetazolamide in the treatment of metabolic alkalosis, *Heart Lung* 20(5):455-459, 1991.

Mays PA: Turning ABGs into child's play, *RN* 58(1):36-40, 1995.

Mclean RM: Magnesium and its therapeutic uses: a review, *Am J Med* 96(1):63-76, 1994.

McMahon MM, Farnell MB, Murray MJ: Nutritional support of critically ill patients, *Mayo Clin Proc* 68:911-920, 1993.

Metheny J: Minimizing respiratory complications of nasoenteric tube feedings: state of the science, *Heart Lung* 22(3):213-223, 1993.

Meyer I: Sodium polystyrene sulfonate: a cation exchange resin used in treating hyperkalemia, *ANNA J* 20(1):93-95, 1993.

Mims B: Interpreting ABGs, *RN* 54(3):42-46, 1991.

Moore EE, Moore FA: Immediate enteral nutrition following multisystem trauma: a decade perspective, *J Am Coll Nutr* 10(6):633-648, 1991.

Narins RG, Emmett M: Simple and mixed acid-base disorders: a practical approach, *Medicine* 59:161, 1980.

National Blood Resource Education Program: *Transfusion therapy guidelines for nurses,* NIH Publication No. 90-2668, 1990.

Nicholson LJ: Declogging small-bore feeding tubes, *J Parenter Enteral Nutr* 11(6):594-597, 1987.

Nussbaum SR: Pathophysiology and management of severe hypercalcemia, *Endocrinol Metab Clin North Am* 22(2):343-362, 1993.

Parrillo J, Bone R, editors: *Critical care medicine: principles of diagnoses & management,* St Louis, 1995, Mosby.

Phipps WJ et al: *Medical-surgical nursing: concepts and clinical practice,* ed 5, St Louis, 1995, Mosby.

Robins EV: Burn shock, *Crit Care Nurs Clin North Am* 2(2):299-307, 1990.

Rose BD: *Clinical physiology of acid-base and electrolyte disorders,* ed 4, New York, 1994, McGraw-Hill Book.

Rubeiz GJ et al: Association of hypomagnesemia and mortality in acutely ill medical patients, *Crit Care Med* 21(2):203-209, 1993.

Rude RK: Magnesium metabolism and deficiency, *Endocrinol Metab Clin North Am* 22(2):377-395, 1993.

Russell J: Successful methods for arterial blood gas interpretation, *Crit Care Nurs* 2(4):14-19, 1991.

Schmitz T: The semi-prone position in ARDS: five case studies, *Crit Care Nurs* 11(5):22-33, 1991.

Seshadri V, Meyer-Tettambel OM: Electrolyte and drug management in nutritional support, *Crit Care Nurs Clin North Am* 5(1):31-36, 1993.

Shapiro B et al: *Clinical application of blood gases,* St Louis, 1989, Mosby.

Shapiro B, Peruzzi W: Arterial blood gases. In Parrillo J, Bone R, editors: *Critical care medicine: principles of diagnoses & management,* St Louis, 1995, Mosby.

Stringfield YN: Back to basics, *Am J Nurs* 93(11):43-44, 1993.

Talbot JM: Guidelines for the scientific review of enteral food products for special medical purposes, *J Parenter Enteral Nutr* 15(3):99S-174S, 1991.

Tasota FJ, Wesmiller SW: Assessing ABG's: maintaining the delicate balance, *Nursing 94* 24(5):34-46, 1994.

Taylor D: Respiratory alkalosis, *Nursing 90* 20(7):52-53, 1990.

Titler MG: Interventions related to surveillance, *Nurs Clin North Am* 27(2):495-503, 1992.

Tso EL, Barish RA: Magnesium: clinical considerations, *J Emerg Med* 10:735-745, 1992.

Vander AJ: *Renal physiology,* ed 4, New York, 1991, McGraw-Hill Book.

Webber KS: Nutritional support. In Swearingen PL, Keen JH, editors: *Manual of critical care nursing: nursing interventions and collaborative management,* ed 3, St Louis, 1995, Mosby.

Weiskittel P: Renal-urinary dysfunctions. In Swearingen PL, Keen JH, editors: *Manual of critical care nursing: nursing interventions and collaborative management,* ed 3, St Louis, 1995, Mosby.

Workman ML: Magnesium and phosphorus: the neglected electrolytes, *AACN Clin Issues* 3(3):655-663, 1992.

Yeates S, Blaufuss J: Managing the patient in diabetic ketoacidosis, *Focus Crit Care* 17(3):240-248, 1990.

Yucha CB: Renal control of calcium, *ANNA J* 20(4):440-444, 1993.

Yucha CB: Renal control of phosphorus and magnesium, *ANNA J* 20(4):447-450, 1993.

Zonszein J: Magnesium and diabetes, *Pract Diabetology* 10(2):1-5, 1991.

# Appendix A: Abbreviations Used in This Manual

**ABA:** American Burn Association
**ABG:** Arterial blood gas
**ACTH:** Adrenocorticotropic hormone
**ADH:** Antidiuretic hormone
**ANF:** Atrial natriuretic factor
**ARDS:** Adult respiratory distress syndrome
**ARF:** Acute renal failure
**ATN:** Acute tubular necrosis
**ATP:** Adenosine triphosphate
**AV:** Atrioventricular
**BEE:** Basal energy expenditure
**BMI:** Body mass index
**BP:** Blood pressure
**bpm:** Beats per minute
**BSA:** Body surface area
**BUN:** Blood urea nitrogen
**$Ca^{2+}$:** Calcium ion
**CAVH:** Continuous arteriovenous hemofiltration
**CBC:** Complete blood cell count
**CHF:** Congestive heart failure
**$Cl^-$:** Chloride ion
**cm $H_2O$:** Centimeters of water
**CNS:** Central nervous system
**CO:** Cardiac output
**$CO_2$:** Carbon dioxide
**COPD:** Chronic obstructive pulmonary disease

**CPR:** Cardiopulmonary resuscitation
**CRF:** Chronic renal failure
**CVA:** Cerebrovasular accident
**CVC:** Central venous catheter
**CVP:** Central venous pressure
**DDAVP:** 1-Deamino-8-D-arginine vasopressin
**DI:** Diabetes insipidus
**DKA:** Diabetic ketoacidosis
**dl:** Deciliter
**DPG:** Diphosphoglycerate
**$D_5W$:** 5% aqueous dextrose solution
**ECF:** Extracellular fluid
**ECV:** Effective circulating volume
**ESRD:** End-stage renal disease
**ECG:** Electrocardiogram
**$Fio_2$:** Fraction of inspired oxygen
**GI:** Gastrointestinal
**$H^+$:** Hydrogen ion
**$H_2CO_3$:** Carbonic acid
**HCl:** Hydrochloric acid
**$HCO_3^-$:** Bicarbonate ion
**Hgb:** Hemoglobin
**HHNK:** Hyperosmolar hyperglycemic nonketotic
**$HPO_4^{2-}$:** Phosphate ion (*also abbreviated* $PO_4^{3-}$)
**HR:** Heart rate
**ICF:** Intracellular fluid
**ICP:** Intracranial pressure
**IDDM:** Insulin-dependent diabetes mellitus
**IM:** Intramuscular
**I&O:** Intake and output
**ISF:** Interstitial fluid
**IU:** International unit
**Iμ U:** International microunit
**IV:** Intravenous
**IVF:** Intravascular fluid
**$K^+$:** Potassium ion
**KCl:** Potassium chloride
**kg:** Kilogram
**L:** Liter
**LCT:** Long-chain triglycerides
**LOC:** Level of consciousness

**MAP:** Mean arterial pressure
**MCT:** Medium-chain triglycerides
**mEq:** Milliequivalent
**mg:** Milligram
**$Mg^{2+}$:** Magnesium ion
**$MgSO_4$:** Magnesium sulfate
**MI:** Myocardial infarction
**ml:** Milliliter
**mm Hg:** Millimeters of mercury
**mOsm:** Milliosmole
**$Na^+$:** Sodium ion
**NaCl:** Sodium chloride
**$NaHCO_3$:** Sodium bicarbonate
**ng:** Nanogram
**NG:** Nasogastric
**$NH_3$:** Ammonia
**$NH_4^+$:** Ammonium ion
**NIDDM:** Non–insulin-dependent diabetes mellitus
**NPO:** Nothing by mouth
**NS:** Normal saline, i.e., isotonic solution of NaCl
**$O_2$:** Oxygen
**OTC:** Over-the-counter
**P:** Phosphorus
**PA:** Pulmonary artery
**$Pa_{CO_2}$:** Partial pressure of carbon dioxide in arterial blood
**$Pa_{O_2}$:** Partial pressure of oxygen in arterial blood
**PADP:** Pulmonary artery diastolic pressure
**PAP:** Pulmonary artery pressure
**PAWP:** Pulmonary artery wedge pressure
**pg:** Picogram
**PO:** By mouth
**$PO_4^{3-}$:** Phosphate ion (*also abbreviated* $HPO_4^{2-}$)
**PRBCs:** Packed red blood cells
**prn:** As needed
**PTH:** Parathyroid hormone
**PVC:** Premature ventricular contractions or peripheral venous
    catheter
**q:** Every
**RBC:** Red blood cell
**RDA:** Recommended daily allowance
**ROM:** Range of motion

**RR:** Respiratory rate
**RTA:** Renal tubular acidosis
**SC:** Subcutaneous
**SIADH:** Syndrome of inappropriate secretion of antidiuretic hormone
**SOB:** Shortness of breath
**stat:** Immediately
**SVR:** Systemic vascular resistance
**TBW:** Total body water
**TCF:** Transcellular fluid
**TNA:** Total nutrient admixture
**TPN:** Total parenteral nutrition
**μg:** Microgram
**μ IU:** Microinternational unit
**VS:** Vital sign
**WBC:** White blood cell

# Appendix B: Glossary

**Acidemia:** Change of pH in arterial blood to <7.40.

**Acidosis:** Abnormal accumulation of acid or loss of base from the body.

**Acids:** Substances that can give up a hydrogen ion.

**Active transport:** The movement of solutes across a cell membrane in the absence of a favorable electrochemical or concentration gradient; requires energy.

**Acute renal failure (ARF):** A sudden loss of renal function that is usually reversible.

**Aldosterone:** A mineralocorticoid hormone released by the adrenal cortex that increases the reabsorption (saving) of sodium and secretion and excretion of potassium and hydrogen by the kidneys.

**Alkalemia:** Increase in arterial pH to >7.40.

**Alkalosis:** Abnormal accumulation of bicarbonate or loss of acid in the body.

**Anaerobic metabolism:** Occurs when there is not enough oxygen available for metabolism and alternate pathways are used, resulting in an accumulation of organic acids (lactic acidosis).

**Analog:** A substance with structure and function similar to another substance.

**Anasarca:** Severe generalized edema.

**Angiotensin:** A polypeptide found in the blood and formed by the action of renin on the $\alpha$-2-globulin, angiotensinogen. *Angiotensin I* is converted to *angiotensin II*. Angiotensin II, a potent vasoconstrictor, acts on the adrenal cortex to stimulate the release of aldosterone.

**Anions:** Ions that develop a negative charge in solution. Examples of the body's most common anions include chloride ion, bicarbonate ion, and phosphate ion. Proteins are another important group of anions.

**Anion gap:** Reflection of the anions in plasma (e.g., phosphates, sulfates, and proteinates) that normally are unmeasured. Anion gap is helpful in the differential diagnosis of metabolic acidosis or mixed acid-base disorders.

**Antidiuretic hormone (ADH):** Produced by the hypothalamus and released by the posterior pituitary gland, it increases reabsorption (saving) of water by the kidneys, allowing excretion of a concentrated urine. In addition, ADH is an arterial vasoconstrictor that increases blood pressure by increasing vascular resistance.

**Anuria:** The production of ≤100 ml of urine in 24 hours.

**Arterial blood gases (ABGs):** Measurement of pH, carbon dioxide tension, and oxygen tension of arterial blood to evaluate acid-base and pulmonary functions.

**Asterixis:** Hand-flapping tremor that occurs with extension of the arm and dorsiflexion of the wrist. It is often seen with metabolic disorders.

**Atrial natriuretic factor (ANF):** Recently identified hormone that is released by the cardiac atria in response to an increased vascular volume. ANF reduces blood pressure and vascular volume.

**Atrial natriuretic peptide (ANP):** Another term for atrial natriuretic factor.

**Azotemia:** Increased retention of metabolic wastes.

**Baroreceptors:** Pressure-sensitive nerve endings located in the carotid sinuses, aortic arch, cardiac atria, and renal vessels, which respond to changes in blood pressure via changes in stretch in the arterial wall, leading to changes in cardiac output, vascular resistance, thirst, and renal handling of sodium and water.

**Bases:** Substances that can take on a hydrogen ion.

**Bicarbonate ($HCO_3^-$):** The body's most important and abundant buffer. It is generated in the kidney and aids in excretion of hydrogen ion.

**Buffers:** Substances that combine with excess acid or base, resulting in a minimally altered pH.

**Capillary membrane:** Separates the intravascular fluid from the interstitial fluid.

**Cardiac output (CO):** Product of heart rate times stroke volume (i.e., the amount of blood moved with each contraction of the left ventricle per minute). Normal value is 4 to 7 L/min for the adult.

**Cations:** Ions that develop a positive charge in solution and are attracted to negative electrons. Examples of the body's most common cations include sodium ions, potassium ions, calcium ions, magnesium ions, and hydrogen ions.

**Cell membrane:** Composed of lipids and protein, this membrane separates intracellular fluid from the interstitial fluid.

**Central venous pressure (CVP):** Measurement of the right atrial pressure and right ventricular end-diastolic pressure via a catheter inserted in or near the right atrium.

**Chronic renal failure (CRF):** An irreversible loss of kidney function, also known as *end-stage renal disease (ESRD).*

**Chvostek's sign:** A signal of tetany occurring with hypocalcemia or hypomagnesemia, it is considered positive when there is unilateral contraction of the facial and eyelid muscles in response to facial nerve percussion.

**Colloid:** In the medical vernacular, colloid is an intravenous fluid that contains solutes *that do not readily* cross the capillary membrane. Dextran, blood, albumin, mannitol, and plasma are all colloids. When combined with water, colloids do not form true solutions.

**Concentration gradient:** The concentration difference between an area of a high concentration and an area of low concentration of the same substance.

**Crystalloid:** In the medical vernacular, crystalloid is an intravenous fluid that contains solutes *that readily* cross the capillary membrane. Examples include dextrose or electrolyte solutions. When combined with water, crystalloids dissolve and form true solutions.

**Diffusion:** Random movement of particles through a solution or gas, in which the particles move from an area of high concentration to an area of low concentration. When diffusion of a particular solute is dependent on the availability of a carrier substance, it is termed *facilitated diffusion.* Diffusion not dependent on a carrier substance is termed *simple diffusion.*

**Edema:** Palpable swelling of the interstitial space that can be either localized or generalized.

**Effective circulating volume (ECV):** The portion of intravascular volume that actually perfuses the tissues. For example, in congestive heart failure intravascular volume increases because of sodium and water retention, yet ECV decreases because of the pooling of blood in the venous circuit.

**Effective osmolality:** Changes in osmolality that will cause water to move from one compartment to another. If a substance has an equal concentration on both sides of the membrane, there is no effective osmolality. *Tonicity* is another term for effective osmolality.

**Electrolytes:** Substances (solutes) that dissociate in solution and conduct an electric current. Electrolytes dissociate into positive ions (cations) and negative ions (anions).

**Epithelial membrane:** Separates interstitial fluid and intravascular fluid from the transcellular fluid and produces transcellular fluid.

**Erythropoietin:** A glycoprotein hormone released by the renal cells in response to low oxygen levels, which stimulates production of red blood cells by the bone marrow.

**Extracellular fluid (ECF):** Fluid found outside the cells, comprising approximately one third of the body's fluid (in the adult).

**Filtration:** Movement of water and solutes from an area of high hydrostatic pressure to an area of low hydrostatic pressure.

**Glomerular filtration rate (GFR):** The volume of fluid crossing the glomerular membrane each minute.

**Hemolysis:** Breakdown of red blood cells that may occur if blood is exposed to a hypotonic solution.

**Homeostasis:** Physiologic balance in which there is relative constancy in the body's environment, maintained by adaptive responses.

**Hydrostatic pressure:** Pressure created by the weight of fluid.

**Hydraulic pressure:** One of the factors that affects the movement of fluid across the capillary membrane. It is a combination of hydrostatic pressure and the pressure created by the pump action of the heart. The terms *hydrostatic pressure* and *hydraulic pressure* are often used interchangeably.

**Hypercapnia:** Increased amounts of carbon dioxide in the blood caused by hypoventilation. It is also known as hypercarbia.

**Hypertonicity:** State in which a solution's effective osmolality is greater than that of the body's fluids.

**Hyperventilation:** Any process resulting in a decreased $Paco_2$.

**Hypervolemia:** Expansion of the extracellular fluid volume. Usually used to describe the expansion of the intravascular portion of the extracellular fluid.

**Hypocapnia:** Decreased amounts of carbon dioxide in the blood caused by hyperventilation. It is also known as hypocarbia.

**Hypotonicity:** State in which a solution's effective osmolality is less than that of the body's fluids.

**Hypoventilation:** Any process resulting in an increased $Paco_2$.

**Hypovolemia:** A reduction in the extracellular fluid volume. Usually used to describe a reduction in the volume of the intravascular portion of the extracellular fluid.

**Insensible fluid:** Imperceptible loss of fluid through the skin or respiratory system via evaporation. Because it is nearly free of electrolytes, insensible fluid loss is considered pure water loss.

**Interstitial fluid (ISF):** The fluid surrounding the cells, including lymph fluid.

**Intracellular fluid (ICF):** Fluid contained within the cells, comprising approximately two thirds of the body's fluid (in the adult).

**Intravascular fluid (IVF):** Fluid contained within the blood vessels (i.e., plasma).

**Isohydric principle:** This principle states that a change in the hydrogen ion concentration will affect the ratio of acids to bases in all buffer systems.

**Isotonic solutions:** Fluids with the same effective osmolality as body fluids.

**Kussmaul's respirations:** Rapid, deep, *sighing* breaths.

**Mean arterial pressure (MAP):** A reflection of the average pressure within the arterial tree throughout the cardiac cycle. The normal value is 70 to 105 mm Hg.

**Metastatic calcifications:** Precipitation and deposition of calcium phosphate in the soft tissue, joints, and arteries, also known as *soft tissue calcifications.*

**Milk-alkali syndrome:** Renal dysfunction and metabolic alkalosis resulting from chronic ingestion of excessive amounts of absorbable alkali (i.e., milk and calcium carbonate).

**Minute ventilation:** Respiratory rate × tidal volume.

**Nonelectrolytes:** Substances that do not dissociate (separate) in solution. Examples include glucose, urea, creatinine, and bilirubin.

**Nonvolatile (fixed) acid:** Any acid that cannot be vaporized and excreted by the lungs.

**Oliguria:** Urinary output of less than 400 ml in 24 hours.

**Oncotic pressure:** Osmotic pressure exerted by protein.

**Osmolality:** Osmotic concentration of body fluids (i.e., the number of dissolved substances per kilogram of water) measured in mOsm/kg of water.

**Osmolarity:** Like osmolality, *osmolarity* is a term used to describe the concentration of fluids; measured in mOsm/L of solution.

**Osmosis:** Movement of water across a semipermeable membrane from an area of lower solute concentration to an area of higher solute concentration.

**Osmotic diuresis:** Increased urine output caused by such substances as mannitol, glucose, or contrast media, which are excreted in the urine and reduce water reabsorption.

**Osmotic pressure:** The pressure that *pulls* water across a semipermeable membrane when the membrane separates two solutions with different concentrations. See *osmosis.*

**Oxygen saturation:** The degree to which hemoglobin is combined with oxygen.

**pH:** Measurement of hydrogen ion concentration in body fluids reflecting one of the following states: normal (7.40), acidic (<7.40), or alkalotic (>7.40).

**Plasma:** The fluid portion of the blood containing water, protein, and electrolytes.

**Polyuria:** Excessive urine output.

**Pulmonary artery pressure (PAP):** Pressure measured in the pulmonary artery. When pulmonary function is normal, it reflects the pressure within the left ventricle at the end of diastole. PAP is used to evaluate left ventricular function and fluid volume. Normal PAP is 20 to 30/8 to 15 mm Hg.

**Pulmonary artery wedge pressure (PAWP):** Measurement of the pulmonary capillary pressure by means of a balloon-tipped catheter passed into the distal pulmonary artery. It provides a more accurate reflection of left ventricular end-diastolic pressure than pulmonary artery pressure. Normal PAWP is 6 to 12 mm Hg.

**Renin:** Proteolytic enzyme produced and released by specialized cells located in the arterioles of the kidney. Renin is released in response to decreased renal perfusion or stimulation of the sympathetic nervous system and is important in the formation of angiotensin.

**Sensible fluid:** Perceptible loss of body fluid (i.e., sweat) via the skin; contains a significant amount of electrolytes.

**Serum:** Plasma minus the fibrinogen and other clotting factors (i.e., the fluid that remains after a blood specimen has been allowed to form a clot).

**Sodium-potassium pump:** A physiologic mechanism present in all body cell membranes that transports sodium from the inside of the cell to the outside and transports potassium from the outside of the cell to the inside. It requires energy and the presence of adequate magnesium.

**Solutes:** Dissolved particles found in body fluids. There are two types: electrolytes and nonelectrolytes.

**Specific gravity:** Measurement of the weight of a substance in relationship to water. Water = 1.000.

**Substrate:** A substance that is acted upon (and changed by) an enzyme during a chemical reaction.

**Syndrome of inappropriate secretion of antidiuretic hormone (SIADH):** A condition in which there is inappropriate hypothalamic production or enhanced action or ectopic production of antidiuretic hormone, resulting in excess water retention.

**Systemic vascular resistance (SVR):** Clinical measurement of the resistance in vessels, which is used to determine workload of the left ventricle (afterload). Normal SVR is 900 to 1200 dynes/sec/cm$^{-5}$.

**Tachypnea:** Increased respiratory rate. It is also called *hyperpnea.*

**Third-space fluid shift:** The loss of extracellular fluid into a normally nonequilibrating space. Although the fluid has not been lost from the body, it is temporarily unavailable to the intracellular fluid or extracellular fluid for its use.

**Tidal volume:** Normal resting volume of ventilation.

**Tonicity:** Another term for *effective osmolality.*

**Transcellular fluid (TCF):** Fluid secreted by epithelial cells. These fluids include cerebrospinal, pericardial, pleural, synovial, and intraocular fluids and digestive secretions.

**Trousseau's sign:** Ischemia-induced carpal spasm that occurs with hypocalcemia and hypomagnesemia. It may be elicited by applying a blood pressure cuff to the upper arm and inflating it past systolic blood pressure for 2 minutes.

**Ventilation-perfusion mismatch:** An inequality in the ratio between ventilation and perfusion that occurs with shunting of venous blood past unventilated alveoli.

**Volatile acid:** An acid that can be vaporized and eliminated by the lungs (i.e., carbon dioxide).

# Appendix C: Effects of Age on Fluid, Electrolyte, and Acid-Base Balance

## Infants and Children

- Relative to their size, infants and children have a greater body surface area (BSA) (both external and internal) than the adult, and thus have a greater potential for fluid loss via the skin and gastrointestinal tract.
- Infants and children have a higher percentage of total body water (TBW) than adults. The greater percentage of the infant's body water is extracellular. As cellular growth occurs, more fluid becomes intracellular.
- Infants have a decreased ability to concentrate their urine, whereas at the same time they have an increased solute load to excrete because of their increased caloric need. These two factors result in a relatively greater obligatory fluid loss, meaning that they must produce a relatively larger volume of urine to excrete their daily load of metabolic wastes.
- The daily intake and output (I&O) for infants (e.g., 650 ml) is equal to approximately half the volume of their extracellular fluid (ECF) (e.g., 1300 ml), as compared with adults, whose daily I&O (e.g., 2500 ml) is approximately one sixth of their ECF (e.g., 15 L). Thus infants can lose a volume equal to their ECF in 2 days, whereas it takes an adult 6 days to do the same.

- Because of an infant's small size and decreased ability to excrete excess fluid, intravenous (IV) fluid administration necessitates caution via use of monitored pumps.
- Infants are less able to compensate for acidosis because of their decreased ability to acidify urine.
- Infants are at increased risk for developing hypernatremia because they are unable to verbalize thirst. Remember that thirst is the body's primary defense against symptomatic hypernatremia.
- Children have an increased incidence and intensity of fever, upper respiratory infections, and gastroenteritis, which can lead to abnormal fluid and electrolyte loss. See Chapter 18 for a discussion of the various fluid and electrolyte imbalances that occur with loss of upper and lower gastrointestinal contents.
- Infants and small children are prone to fluid volume deficit caused by a combination of the factors listed previously. Unfortunately, some of the common indicators of fluid volume deficit are less reliable in the infant or small child. Infants are unable to verbalize thirst, although their cries may become increasingly high-pitched. Skin turgor also may be a less reliable sign. Skin turgor may appear normal in the obese infant because of increased subcutaneous fat, or it may appear abnormal in the adequately hydrated but undernourished infant. Irritability is an early indicator of hypovolemia. Sunken fontanels, a traditional indicator of dehydration, does not occur until there has been moderate to severe fluid loss.

## The Older Adult

- Weight (body fat) tends to increase with advancing age, thus the percentage of TBW decreases. Recall that fat cells contain little water. The percentage of TBW increases in the emaciated individual who has lost significant body fat.
- Renal function decreases with advancing age. Glomerular filtration rate drops; thus the older adult is less likely to compensate for an increased metabolic load. There is also a reduction in the ability to concentrate urine, resulting in greater obligatory water losses. The older adult must produce a larger volume of urine to excrete the same amount of metabolic waste as the younger adult.
- In the older adult, the kidneys are less able to compensate for an acid load, resulting in decreased ammonia formation.

(Ammonia produced by the renal tubular cell diffuses into the lumen of the tubule and combines with hydrogen to form ammonium, which is then excreted in the urine. In this way, ammonia acts as a urinary buffer, allowing increased excretion of hydrogen ions.) Normally, ammonia production increases in the presence of an acid load.

- Decreased respiratory function also reduces the older adult's ability to compensate for acid-base imbalance. The older adult is also more likely to develop hypoxemia.

- There is a reduction in the secretion of hydrochloric acid (HCl) by the stomach, which may affect the individual's ability to tolerate certain foods. The older adult is especially prone to constipation because of decreased gastrointestinal tract motility. Limited fluid intake, a restricted diet, and a reduced level of physical activity may contribute to the development of constipation. Excessive or inappropriate use of laxatives may lead to problems with diarrhea.

- As the skin ages, there is a reduction in insensible and sensible water loss secondary to decreased skin hydration and decreased functioning of the sweat glands. Thus the skin is less efficient in cooling the body, and the skin tends to be dry. In addition, skin turgor is a less reliable indicator of fluid status as a result of decreased skin elasticity.

- Older adults are at increased risk for developing hypernatremia because they have a less sensitive thirst center and may have problems with obtaining fluids (e.g., impaired mobility) or expressing their desire for fluids (e.g., the individual with expressive asphasia). Thirst is the body's primary defense against symptomatic hypernatremia.

# Appendix D: Laboratory Tests Discussed in This Manual (Normal Values)*

| Complete Blood Cell Count | Adult Normal Values |
| --- | --- |
| Hemoglobin | Male: 14-18 g/dl |
| | Female: 12-16 g/dl |
| Hematocrit | Male: 40%-54% |
| | Female: 37%-47% |
| Red blood cell count | Male: 4.5-6 million/µl |
| | Female: 4-5.5 million/µl |
| White blood cell count | 4500-11,000/µl |
| Neutrophils | 54%-75% (3000-7500/µl) |
| Band neutrophils | 3%-8% (150-700/µl) |
| Lymphocytes | 25%-40% (1500-4500/µl) |
| Monocytes | 2%-8% (100-500/µl) |
| Eosinophils | 1%-4% (50-400/µl) |
| Basophils | 0%-1% (25-100/µl) |
| Platelet count | 150,000-400,000/µl |

*Normal values may vary significantly with different laboratory methods of testing.

| Serum, Plasma, and Whole Blood Chemistry | Normal Values |
|---|---|
| ACTH | 8 AM-10 AM <100 pg/ml |
| ADH | 0-2 pg/ml/serum osmolality <285 mOsm/kg; |
| | 2-12 pg/ml/serum osmolality >290 mOsm/kg |
| Albumin | 3.5-5.5 g/dl |
| Aldosterone | Male: 6-22 ng/dl |
| | Female: 4-31 ng/dl |
| Ammonia | Adult: 15-110 µg/dl |
| | Child: 56-80 µg/dl |
| | Newborn: 90-150 µg/dl |
| Amylase | 60-180 Somogyi U/dl |
| Base, total | 145-160 mEq/L |
| Bicarbonate | 22-26 mEq/L |
| Bilirubin | Total: 0.3-1.4 mg/dl |
| ABGs | |
| pH | 7.35-7.45 |
| $Paco_2$ | 35-45 mm Hg |
| $Pao_2$ | 80-95 mm Hg |
| $O_2$ saturation | 95%-99% |
| Blood urea nitrogen | 6-20 mg/dl |
| Calcitonin | <100 pg/ml |
| Calcium | 8.5-10.5 mg/dl; 4.3-5.3 mEq/L |
| Chloride | 95-108 mEq/L |
| Cortisol | 8 AM-10 AM: 5-25 µg/dl |
| | 4 PM-12 AM (midnight): 2-18 µg/dl |
| $CO_2$ content (total $CO_2$) | 22-28 mEq/L |

*ACTH,* Adrenocorticotropic hormone; *ADH,* antidiuretic hormone; *ABGs,* arterial blood gases; *Paco₂,* partial pressure of carbon dioxide in arterial blood; *Pao₂,* partial pressure of oxygen in arterial blood; *O₂,* oxygen; *CO₂,* carbon dioxide; *CPK,* creatinine phosphokinase.

| Serum, Plasma, and Whole Blood Chemistry | Normal Values |
|---|---|
| CPK | Male: 55-170 U/L |
| | Female: 30-135 U/L |
| Creatinine | 0.6-1.5 mg/dl |
| Creatinine clearance | Male: 107-141 ml/min |
| | Female: 87-132 ml/min |
| Globulins, total | 1.5-3.5 g/dl |
| Glucose, fasting | True glucose: 65-110 mg/dl |
| | All sugars: 80-120 mg/dl |
| Glucose, 2-hr postprandial | <145 mg/dl |
| Glucose tolerance | Fasting: 65-110 mg/dl |
|   Intravenous | 5 min: maximum 250 mg/dl |
| | 60 min: decrease |
| | 2 hr: <120 mg/dl |
| | 3 hr: 65-110 mg/dl |
|   Oral | Fasting: 65-110 mg/dl |
| | 30 min: <155 mg/dl |
| | 1 hr: <165 mg/dl |
| | 2 hr: <120 mg/dl |
| | 3 hr: ≤65-110 mg/dl |
| 17-OCHS | Male: 7-19 μg/dl |
| | Female: 9-21 μg/dl |
| Insulin | 11-240 μ IU/ml |
| | 4-24 μ U/ml |
| Iron | Total: 60-200 μg/dl |
| | Male, average: 125 μg/dl |
| | Female, average: 100 μg/dl |
| | Elderly: 60-80 μg/dl |
| Ketone bodies | 2-4 μg/dl |

| Serum, Plasma, and Whole Blood Chemistry | Normal Values |
|---|---|
| Lactic acid | Arterial: 0.5-1.6 mEq/L |
| | Venous: 1.5-2.2 mEq/L |
| Magnesium | 1.8-3 mg/dl |
| | 1.5-2.5 mEq/L |
| Osmolality | 280-300 mOsm/kg |
| Parathyroid hormone | <2000 pg/ml |
| Phosphatase, acid | 0-1.1 U/ml (Bodansky) |
| | 1-4 U/ml (King-Armstrong) |
| | 0.13-0.63 U/ml (Bessey-Lowery) |
| Phosphatase alkaline | 1.5-4.5 U/dl (Bodansky) |
| | 4-13 U/dl (King-Armstrong) |
| | 0.8-2.3 U/ml (Bessey-Lowery) |
| Phosphorus | 2.5-4.5 mg/dl; 1.7-2.6 mEq/L |
| Potassium | 3.5-5 mEq/L |
| Renin | Normal sodium intake |
| |    Supine (4-6 hr): 0.5-1.6 ng/ml/hr |
| |    Sitting (4 hr): 1.8-3.6 ng/ml/hr |
| | Low sodium intake |
| |    Supine (4-6 hr): 2.2-4.4 ng/ml/hr |
| |    Sitting (4 hr): 4-8.1 ng/ml/hr |
| Sodium | 135-145 mEq/L |
| Thyroid stimulating hormone | 4.6 $\mu$ U/ml |
| Urea clearance | |
| Serum/24-hr urine | 64-99 ml/min (maximum clearance) |
| Uric acid | 41-65 ml/min (standard clearance) |
| | Male: 2.1-7.5 mg/dl |
| | Female: 2-6.6 mg/dl |

| Urine Chemistry | Normal Values |
|---|---|
| Albumin | |
|   Random | Negative |
|   24-hr | 10-100 mg/24 hr |
| Amylase | |
|   2-hr | 35-260 (Somogyi) U/hr |
|   24-hr | 80-5000 U/24 hr |
| Bilirubin | |
|   Random | Negative: 0.02 mg/dl |
| Calcium | |
|   Random | 1 + turbidity; 10 mg/dl |
|   24-hr | 50-300 mg/24 hr |
| Creatinine | |
|   24-hr | Male: 20-26 mg/kg/24 hr |
| | Female: 14-22 mg/kg/24 hr |
| Creatinine clearance | Male: 107-141 ml/min |
| | Female: 87-132 ml/min |
| Glucose | |
|   Random | Negative: 15 mg/dl |
|   24-hr | 130 mg/24 hr |
| Ketone | |
|   24-hr | Negative: 0.3-2 mg/dl |
| Osmolality | |
|   Random | 350-700 mOsm/kg |
|   24-hr | 300-900 mOsm/kg |
|   Physiologic range | 50-1400 mOsm/kg |
| pH | |
|   Random | 4.6-8 |
| Phosphorus | |
|   24-hr | 0.9-1.3 g; 0.2-0.6 mEq/L |

| Urine Chemistry | Normal Values |
|---|---|
| Protein | |
| Random | Negative: 2-8 mg/dl |
| 24-hr | 40-150 mg |
| Sodium | |
| Random | 50-130 mEq/L |
| 24-hr | 40-220 mEq/L |
| Specific gravity | |
| Random | 1.010-1.020 |
| After fluid restriction | 1.025-1.035 |
| Sugar | |
| Random | Negative |
| Urea clearance | |
| 24-hr | 64-99 ml/min (maximum) |
| | 41-65 ml/min (standard) |
| Urea nitrogen | |
| 24-hr | 6-17 g |

# Index

## A

Abbreviations, 270-273
Abnormal reflexes, 34
Acid-base balance
  blood gas values in, 142, 143*t*
    arterial analysis, 142, 144-145*t*, 148
    arterial-venous difference, 149, 152
    mixed venous, 149
  buffer system responses in
    buffers, 140-141
    renal, 141
    respiratory, 141
  diet for correcting, 264
  effects of age on, 281-283
  general guidelines for, 150-151*t*
  quick assessment guide to, 146-149*t*
  tests in evaluating, 40-42, 40*t*, *41, 43*, 44
Acid-base disturbances, 79
  in acute adrenal insufficiency, 216-217
  in acute pancreatitis, 230-232
  in cardiogenic shock, 220
  case studies of mixed, 186-189, 187*t*
  in congestive heart failure, 219
  in diabetes mellitus, 211, 215
  in diabetic ketoacidosis, 205-206
  in hyperosmolar hyperglycemic nonketotic syndrome, 207, 209

Acid-base disturbances—cont'd
  with loss of lower gastrointestinal contents, 200
  with loss of upper gastrointestinal contents, 196
  as postoperative surgical disturbances, 203
  in pulmonary edema, 219
  in renal failure, 226-229, *227, 228*
  in syndrome of inappropriate secretion of antidiuretic hormone, 215
Acidemia, 141
Acidosis
  metabolic, 236, 237, 244
  respiratory, 237, 244, 264
Active transport, 9-10
Acute adrenal insufficiency, 216
  and fluid, electrolyte, and acid-base disturbances, 216-217
Acute tubular necrosis (ATN), 221
Addison's disease, 136
Adrenal insufficiency, 36
Adult respiratory distress syndrome (ARDS), 156
Age
  and body fluids, 3, 4*t*
  effects of, on fluid, electrolyte, and acid-base balance, 281-283
Albumin, 247
Alcoholism
  as cause of hypomagnesemia, 131
  treatment of ketoacidosis related to, 174
Aldosterone, 19
Alkalizing agents in managing chronic metabolic acidosis, 177
Alkalosis
  hypokalemic, 235
  metabolic, 236
  respiratory, 118-119, 120, 236, 244

Note: Page numbers in *italics* indicate figures; Page numbers followed by a *t* indicate tables.

Aluminum hydroxide antacids for hypocalcemia, 110
Ammonium and acid-base balance, 141
Anasarca. *See* Edema formation
Anion gap, 41-42, *41*
  in metabolic acidosis, 172-173, 173*t*
Anions, 9
  in body fluids, 4, 5*t,* 6
Anorexia, 34
Anthropometric data, 246
Antidiuretic hormone (ADH), 20, *18*
  medications that alter action of, *22*
  and thirst, 21-22
Anuria, 25
Arterial blood gas (ABG), 40
  in acute metabolic alkalosis, 181
  in acute respiratory acidosis, 155
  in acute respiratory alkalosis, 166
  in chronic metabolic acidosis, 175
  in chronic metabolic alkalosis, 184
  in chronic respiratory acidosis, 161
  in chronic respiratory alkalosis, 168
  in hyperkalemia, 103
  in hypervolemia, 68-69
  in hypovolemia, 53
  in metabolic acidosis, 172
  normal ranges for, 40*t*
Ascites, 234
Assessment
  for acute metabolic acidosis, 170, *171,* 172
  for acute respiratory acidosis, 153-155, *154*
  for acute respiratory alkalosis, 165-166
  for chronic metabolic acidosis, 175
  for chronic metabolic alkalosis, 183-184
  for chronic respiratory acidosis, 160-161, *161*
  for chronic respiratory alkalosis, 168
  for hypercalcemia, 113-114
  for hyperkalemia, 102-103
  for hypermagnesemia, 136-137
  for hyperphosphatemia, 125-126
  for hypocalcemia, 108-109
  for hypomagnesemia, 131-132
  for hypophosphatemia, 119-121
Atrial natriuretic factor (ANF), *18,* 19-20
Atrial natriuretic peptide, *18,* 19
Azotemia, 79

**B**

Bicarbonate and acid-base balance, 141
Bile in gastrointestinal disorders, 198

Bilirubin in body fluids, 6
Biochemical data, 247-250
Blood gas values, 142, 143*t*
  arterial analysis, 142, 144-145*t,* 148
  arterial-venous difference, 149, 152
  mixed venous, 149
Blood pressure, 31-32
Blood urea nitrogen (BUN)
  in hypervolemia, 68-69
  in hypovolemia, *52,* 52-53
Body fluids
  composition of, 3-4, 4*t,* 5*t,* 6
  concentration of, 11-13
  gains, 23-24, 23*t*
  losses, 23*t,* 24-26
Body Mass Index (BMI), 247
Body temperature, 30-31
Bowel obstruction in gastrointestinal disorders, 199-200
Brain cell volume, defense of, 22
Breathing pattern, ineffective, in hypocalcemia, 112
Buffers, 140-141
Buffer system responses
  buffers, 140-141
  renal, 141
  respiratory, 141
Burns, 237-240
  American Burn Association classification system for, 241*t*
  characteristics of wound depth, 238*t*
  estimation of injury, *240*
  factors determining severity of, *242*
  fluid, electrolyte, and acid-base disturbances with, 242, 244
  formulas used in estimating fluid requirements in, 243*t*
  full-thickness, 238
  partial-thickness, 238
  rule of nines in, *239*

**C**

Calcitonin, 114-115
Calcium
  foods high in, *111*
  for hypocalcemia, 109-110, 110*t*
  relationship between ionized, and plasma pH, 107-108
Calcium acetate for hypocalcemia, 110
Calcium balance disorders, 107-108
  hypercalcemia as, 113
    assessment of, 113-114
    collaborative management of, 114-115
    diagnostic tests for, 114

Calcium balance disorders—cont'd
  hypercalcemia as—cont'd
    nursing diagnoses and
        interventions for, 115
    patient-family teaching guidelines
        for, 116-117
  hypocalcemia as, 108
    assessment of, 108-109
    collaborative management of,
        109-110, 110*t*
    diagnostic tests for, 109
    nursing diagnoses and
        interventions for, 110-112
    patient-family teaching guidelines
        for, 112-113
Calories, distribution of, 249
Calorimetry, indirect, 249
Capillary membranes, 8
Carbohydrates
  in enteral products, 253
  in parenteral solution, 261
Carbon dioxide content, 40-41
Cardiac disorders
  cardiogenic shock as, 219-220
    fluid, electrolyte, and acid-base
        disturbances in, 220
  congestive heart failure as, 218
    fluid, electrolyte, and acid-base
        disturbances in, 219
  pulmonary edema as, 218
    fluid, electrolyte, and acid-base
        disturbances in, 219
Cardiac output, 31
  decreased, in hypocalcemia,
      112
Cardiogenic shock, 219-220
  fluid, electrolyte, and acid-base
      disturbances in, 220
Cardiovascular system, 32-33
Catheter irrigants, 29
Cations, 9
  in body fluids, 4
Cell membranes, 8
Cells, 3
  effect of osmotic pressure of, *12*
Cell walls, 9
Central venous pressure (CVP), 30
Chest physiotherapy for management
    of respiratory acidosis, 162
Chest x-ray
  in assessing acute respiratory
      acidosis, 155
  in assessing chronic respiratory
      acidosis, 162
  in assessing hypervolemia, 69
Chloride, 4

Chvostek's sign, positive, 34
  in assessing hyperphospatemia, 128
  in assessing hypocalcemia, 108
Cirrhosis, 234
  Laennec's, 233
Clinical assessment, 28
  daily weights, 28
Clinical hypertonicity, 13
Clinical hypotonicity, 12-13
Collaborative management
  for acute metabolic acidosis,
      173-174
  for acute metabolic alkalosis,
      181-182
  for acute respiratory acidosis, 155
  for acute respiratory alkalosis, 167
  for chronic metabolic acidosis, 177
  for chronic metabolic alkalosis,
      184-185
  for chronic respiratory acidosis, 162
  for chronic respiratory alkalosis, 169
  for hypercalcemia, 114-115
  for hyperkalemia, 103-104
  for hypermagnesemia, 137-138
  for hypernatremia, 93
  for hyperphosphatemia, 126-127, 127*t*
  for hypocalcemia, 109-110, 110*t*
  for hypokalemia, 97, 99
  for hypomagnesemia, 133
  for hyponatremia, 89
  for hypophosphatemia, *121,* 121-122
Colloids, 86
Confusion, 34
Congestive heart failure, fluid, electro-
    lyte, and acid-base disturbances
    in, 219
Cortisone, 114
Creatinine, 44
  in body fluids, 6
Creatinine-height index, 248
Crohn's disease, 199
Crying and fluid loss, 26
Crystalloid solutions, 81

**D**

Diabetes insipidus, 36, 211, 212-214*t*
  fluid, electrolyte, and acid-base
      disturbances in, 211, 215
Diabetic ketoacidosis (DKA), 119,
    204-205
  treatment of, 174
Diagnostic tests
  for acute metabolic acidosis,
      172-173, 173*t*
  for acute metabolic alkalosis, 181

Diagnostic tests—cont'd
for acute respiratory acidosis, 155
for acute respiratory alkalosis,
166-167
for chronic metabolic acidosis, 175,
177
for chronic metabolic alkalosis, 184
for chronic respiratory acidosis,
161-162
for chronic respiratory alkalosis,
168
for hypercalcemia, 114
for hyperkalemia, 103
for hypermagnesemia, 137
for hypernatremia, 92-93
for hyperphosphatemia, 126
for hypervolemia, 68-69
for hypocalcemia, 109
for hypokalemia, 97, *98*
for hypomagnesemia, 132-133
for hyponatremia, 89
for hypophosphatemia, 121
for hypovolemia, *52,* 52-53
Diarrhea, 26
in gastrointestinal disorders, 198
osmotic, *197,* 198-199
potential causes of, *197*
secretory, *197,* 199
Diet; *see also* Nutrition
for correcting acid-base balance,
264
for electrolyte imbalances, 263-264
for hepatic failure, 249
for hyperkalemia, 263
for hypermagnesemia, 264
for hypernatremia, 263
for hyperphosphatemia, 264
for hypervolemia, 263-264
for hypokalemia, 264
for hypomagnesemia, 264
for hyponatremia, 263
for hypophosphatemia, 264
for hypovolemia, 263
Diffusion, 8-9
facilitated, 9
factors that increase, *9*
simple, 9
Dilutional hyponatremia, 200
Diuretic therapy, 36
complications of, 75-77, 80
for edema formation, 75, 78-79*t*
Draining fistulas, 29
Drug screen in acute respiratory
acidosis, 155
Dysrhythmias, 33

**E**

Edema, 32, 235
formation, 73-74, *74*
assessment of, 74-75
collaborative management of, 75
complications of diuretic therapy,
75, 78-80
diuretic therapy, 75, 76-77*t*
generalized, 74
potential fluid, electrolyte, and
acid-base disturbances in,
219
sacral, 74
Effective circulating volume
(ECV), 14
changes in, 15
reduction in, 234-235
Effective osmolality, 12
Effective osmoles, 12
Electrocardiogram (ECG), in
diagnosing
acute metabolic alkalosis, 179, 181
acute respiratory alkalosis, 167
chronic respiratory acidosis, 162
diagnosing acidosis, 173
hyperkalemia, 103
hypocalcemia, 109
Electrolytes
in body fluids, 4, 5*t,* 6
diet for imbalances, 263-264
disturbances
in acute adrenal insufficiency,
216-217
in acute pancreatitis, 230-232
in cardiogenic shock, 220
in congestive heart failure, 219
in diabetes mellitus, 211, 215
in diabetic ketoacidosis, 205-206
and diuretic therapy, 78-79
in hyperosmolar hyperglycemic
nonketotic syndrome, 207,
209
with loss of lower gastrointestinal
contents, 200
with loss of upper gastrointestinal
contents, 196
as postoperative surgical
disturbances, 203
in pulmonary edema, 219
in renal failure, 226-229, *227, 228*
in syndrome of inappropriate
secretion of antidiuretic
hormone, 215
effects of age on, 281-283
tests to evaluate balance, 39

Endocrinologic disorders
  acute adrenal insufficiency as, 216
    fluid, electrolyte, and acid-base
      disturbances in, 216-217
  diabetes insipidus as, 211, 212-214*t*
    fluid, electrolyte, and acid-base
      disturbances in, 211, 215
  diabetic ketoacidosis as, 204-205
    fluid, electrolyte, and acid-base
      disturbances in, 205
  hyperosmolar hyperglycemic
      nonketotic syndrome as,
      206-207, 208-210*t*
    fluid, electrolyte, and acid-base
      disturbances in, 207, 211
  syndrome of inappropriate secretion
      of antidiuretic hormone as,
      215
    fluid, electrolyte, and acid-base
      disturbances in, 215
Enteral nutrition, 250-253
  feeding tubes and sites in, 251-252
  formulations in, 254-255*t*
  infusion rates in, 252, 252*t*
  managing complications in, 256,
      257-259*t*
  products in, 253, 254-255*t*, 255
Epithelial membranes, 8
Erythrocytes, 7
Erythropoietin, production of, in
      kidney, *222*
Etidronate, 114
Excessive sweating, 29
Extracellular fluid (ECF), 14
  in body fluids, 6-8
  osmolality of, 11
    regulation of, 20-22
  sodium in maintaining, 87

## F

Facilitated diffusion, 9
Fat cells and body fluids, 3, 4*t*
Fats
  in enteral products, 255
  in parenteral solution, 261
Female gender and body fluids, 3, 4*t*
Fiber in enteral products, 253
Filtration, 10
Fluid balance
  effects of age on, 281-283
  factors affecting, 250
Fluid balance disorders
  edema formation as, 73-74, *74*
    assessment of, 74-75

Fluid balance disorders—cont'd
  edema formation as—cont'd
    collaborative management of, 75
    complications of diuretic therapy,
        75, 78-80
    diuretic therapy, 75, 76-77*t*
  hypervolemia as, 68
    assessment of, 68
    collaborative management of, 69
    diagnostic tests for, 68-69
    nursing diagnosis and interven-
        tions, 70-72, *70*
    patient-family teaching guidelines
        for, 72-73
  hypovolemia as, 49, 50*t*
    assessment of, 49, 51, 51*t*
    collaborative management of,
        53-55, 56-59*t*, 60-63*t*, 64*t*
    diagnostic tests for, *52*, 52-53
    nursing diagnoses and
        intervention, 65-67
    patient-family teaching guidelines
        for, 67
  intravenous fluid therapy in, *80*,
      80-81
    commonly prescribed, 81, 86
Fluid balance disturbances
  in acute adrenal insufficiency,
      216-217
  in acute pancreatitis, 230-232
  in cardiogenic shock, 220
  in congestive heart failure, 219
  in diabetes mellitus, 211, 215
  in diabetic ketoacidosis, 205-206
  in hyperosmolar hyperglycemic
      nonketotic syndrome, 207,
      209
  with loss of lower gastrointestinal
      contents, 200
  with loss of upper gastrointestinal
      contents, 196
  as postoperative surgical
      disturbances, 203
  in pulmonary edema, 219
  in renal failure, 226-229, *227*, *228*
  in syndrome of inappropriate
      secretion of antidiuretic
      hormone, 215
Fluid compartments in body fluids, 6-8,
    *7*
Fluid gains
  oral fluids in, 24
  oxidative metabolism in, 23-24
  solid foods in, 24
  therapy for, 24

Fluid losses
  gastrointestinal tract, 26
  kidneys, 24-25
  lungs, 26
  skin, 25
  third-space, 26
Fluids
  alterations in volume, 234-235
  management of, in chronic metabolic
      alkalosis, 184
  tests to evaluate status, 35-39
Fluid therapy, 24
Fluid volume deficit
  in acute pancreatitis, 230-231
  in cardiogenic shock, 220
  in diabetes insipidus, 211
  in diabetic ketoacidosis, 205
  in hyperosmolar hyperglycemic
      nonketotic syndrome,
      207
  in hyponatremia, 90
  in hypovolemia, 65-66
Fluid volume excess
  in cardiogenic shock, 220
  in congestive heart failure,
      219
  in hypervolemia, 70-71
  in pulmonary edema, 219
Foods; see Nutrition
Free water loss, 36
Full-thickness burns, 238

**G**

Gallium nitrate, 115
Gas exchange, impaired, in
      hypervolemia, 71-72
Gastric juices in gastrointestinal
      disorders, 195
Gastric suction in gastrointestinal
      disorders, 195-196
Gastrointestinal contents
  loss of lower, 197-198
    fluid, electrolyte, and acid-base
        disturbances with, 200
  loss of upper, 193
    fluid, electrolyte, and acid-base
        disturbances with, 196
Gastrointestinal disorders, 193-200,
      194t
  bile in, 198
  bowel obstruction in, 199-200
  diarrhea in, 198-199
  gastric juices in, 195
  gastric suction in, 195-196
  intestinal secretions in, 198

Gastrointestinal disorders—cont'd
  loss of lower contents, 197-198
    potential fluid, electrolyte, and
        acid-base disturbances, 200
  loss of upper contents, 193
    potential fluid, electrolyte, and
        acid-base disturbances
        with, 196
  pancreatic juice in, 198
  saliva in, 193, 195
Gastrointestinal secretions, volume and
      composition of, 193, 194t
Gastrointestinal system, 34
Gastrointestinal tract
  and fluid loss, 26
  in maintaining fluid and electrolyte
      balance, 193
Generalized edema, 74
Glucosuria, 11

**H**

Harris and Benedict equation,
      248-249
Heart rate/pulses, 31
Height, 246
Hematocrit, 36
  in hypervolemia, 68-69
  in hypovolemia, 52-53
Hemodialysis in management of
      chronic metabolic acidosis,
      177
Hemodynamic measurements
  in hyponatremia, 88
  in hypovolemia, 49, 51
Hemodynamic monitoring, 29-30, 30t
Hepatic failure, 233-234
  diet for, 249
  potential fluid, electrolyte, and
      acid-base disturbances,
      234-236
Hepatorenal syndrome, 233
Hepatotoxic potential, drugs with, *234*
Homeostasis, 23
Hydrostatic pressure, 10
Hyperadrenocorticism, 183-184
Hypercalcemia, 113
  assessment of, 113-114
  collaborative management of,
      114-115
  diagnostic tests for, 114
  nursing diagnoses and interventions
      for, 115
  patient-family teaching guidelines
      for, 116-117
Hyperglycemia, 36, 204

Hyperkalemia, 78-79
  in acute adrenal insufficiency, 216
  assessment of, 102-103
  in burns, 242
  collaborative management of, 103-104
  in diabetic ketoacidosis, 205
  diagnostic tests for, 103
  diet for, 263
  and hepatic failure, 235
  nursing diagnoses and interventions for, 104-105
  patient-family teaching guidelines for, 106
  as postoperative surgical disturbances, 203
  in renal failure, 226
Hypermagnesemia
  assessment of, 136-137
  collaborative management of, 137-138
  diagnostic tests for in, 137
  diet for, 264
  nursing diagnoses and interventions for in, 138-139
  patient-family teaching guidelines for, 139
  in renal failure, 229
Hypernatremia, 87, 91
  assessment of, 91-92
  collaborative management of, 93
  in diabetes insipidus, 211, 215
  in diabetic ketoacidosis, 205
  diagnostic tests for, 92-93
  diet for, 263
  nursing diagnoses and interventions for, 93-94
  patient-family teaching guidelines for, 94
Hyperosmolar hyperglycemic nonketotic syndrome, 206-207, 208-210*t*
  potential fluid, electrolyte, and acid-base disturbances, 207, 211
Hyperparathyroidism, 113
Hyperphosphatemia, 125
  assessment of, 125-126
  collaborative management of, 126-127, 127*t*
  in diabetic ketoacidosis, 205
  diagnostic tests for, 126
  diet for, 264
  nursing diagnoses and interventions for, 127-129

Hyperphosphatemia—cont'd
  patient-family teaching guidelines for, 129
  in renal failure, 228
Hypertonic solutions, 12
Hyperuricemia, 77, 80
Hyperventilation, 168
Hypervolemia, 68
  assessment of, 68
  in burns, 242
  collaborative management of, 69
  diagnostic tests for, 68-69
  diet for, 263-264
  nursing diagnosis and interventions, 70-72, *70*
  patient-family teaching guidelines for, 72-73
  in renal failure, 226
  in syndrome of inappropriate secretion of antidiuretic hormone, 215
Hypoalbuminemia, 235
Hypocalcemia, 108, 125
  in acute pancreatitis, 232
  assessment of, 108-109
  in burns, 244
  collaborative management of, 109-110, 110*t*
  diagnostic tests for, 109
  and hepatic failure, 235
  nursing diagnoses and interventions for, 110-112
  patient-family teaching guidelines for, 112-113
  in renal failure, 228-229
Hypocalcemic tetany, 168
Hypocapnia, 165
Hypochloremia in diabetic ketoacidosis, 206
Hypokalemia, 78, 96
  in acute pancreatitis, 232
  assessment of, 96-97
  in burns, 242
  collaborative management of, 97, 99
  in congestive heart failure, 219
  in diabetic ketoacidosis, 205
  diagnostic tests for, 97, *98*
  diet for, 264
  in gastrointestinal disorders, 196, 200
  and hepatic failure, 235
  in hyperosmolar hyperglycemic nonketotic syndrome, 207
  nursing diagnoses and interventions for, 99-101

Hypokalemia—cont'd
  patient-family teaching guidelines
    for, 101-102
  in pulmonary edema, 219
  in renal failure, 228
Hypokalemic alkalosis, 235
Hypomagnesemia, 79, 96, 131
  in acute pancreatitis, 232
  assessment of, 131-132
  collaborative management of, 133
  in diabetic ketoacidosis, 205
  diagnostic tests for, 132-133
  diet for, 264
  in gastrointestinal disorders, 196,
    200
  and hepatic failure, 235
  in hyperosmolar hyperglycemic
    nonketotic syndrome, 207
  nursing diagnoses and interventions
    for, 133-135
  patient-family teaching guidelines
    for, 136
Hyponatremia, 52-53, 79, 88
  in acute adrenal insufficiency, 217
  in acute pancreatitis, 232
  assessment of, 88-89
  in burns, 242
  in cardiogenic shock, 220
  collaborative management of, 89
  in congestive heart failure, 219
  in diabetic ketoacidosis, 205
  diagnostic tests for, 89
  diet for, 263
  dilutional, 200
  with expanded extracellular fluid
    volume, 90
  in gastrointestinal disorders, 196,
    200
  and hepatic failure, 235
  in hyperosmolar hyperglycemic
    nonketotic syndrome, 207
  nursing diagnoses and interventions
    for, 90-91
  patient-family teaching guidelines
    for, 91
  in pulmonary edema, 219
  with reduced extracellular fluid
    volume, 89-90
  in renal failure, 226
  in syndrome of inappropriate
    secretion of antidiuretic
    hormone, 215
Hypophosphatemia, 119
  assessment of, 119-121
  in burns, 244
  in chronic respiratory alkalosis, 169

Hypophosphatemia—cont'd
  collaborative management of, *121,*
    121-122
  in diabetic ketoacidosis, 205
  diagnostic tests for, 121
  diet for, 264
  and hepatic failure, 236
  in hyperosmolar hyperglycemic
    nonketotic syndrome, 207
  nursing diagnoses and interventions
    for, 122-124
  patient-family teaching guidelines
    for, 124-125
Hypoproteinemia, 237
Hypotonic solutions, 12
Hypovolemia, 49, 50*t*
  in acute adrenal insufficiency, 216
  in acute pancreatitis, 231
  assessment of, 49, 51, 51*t*
  in burns, 242
  collaborative management of, 53-55,
    56-59*t*, 60-63*t*, 64*t*
  diagnostic tests for, *52,* 52-53
  diet for, 263
  in gastrointestinal disorders, 196,
    200
  nursing diagnoses and intervention,
    65-67
  patient-family teaching guidelines
    for, 67
  in renal failure, 226
Hypovolemic shock, 49
  restoration of tissue perfusion in, 55,
    56-59*t*, 60-63*t*

**I**

Ileostomy, 197
Indirect calorimetry, 249
Ineffective osmoles, 12
Insensible fluid, 25
Intake and output, 29
Integument, 32
Interstitial fluid (ISF), 36
  in body fluids, 6
Intestinal secretions in gastrointestinal
    disorders, 198
Intracellular fluid (ICF), 14
  in body fluids, 6
Intravascular fluid (IVF), 14
  in body fluids, 6-7
Intravascular space (IVS), 11
Intravenous (IV) fluids
  commonly prescribed, 81, 86
  for management of respiratory
    acidosis, 162

Intravenous (IV) fluids—cont'd
    therapy, *80,* 80-81
        commonly prescribed, 81, 86
        for hypovolemia, 53-55
Isotonic fluid loss, 36
Isotonic solutions, 12

## J

Jugular venous distention, assessment
    of, 32-33

## K

Ketoacidosis, 172
Ketones, 204
Kidneys
    in acid-base balance, 42
    and fluid losses, 24-25
    functions of, *222*
    in potassium balance regulation, 96
Kussmaul's respirations, 205

## L

Laboratory assessment
    of anion gap, 41-42
    of arterial blood gases, 40
    of carbon dioxide content, 40-41
    of creatinine, 44
    of electrolyte balance, 39
    of hematocrit, 36
    of lactic acid, 44
    of serum albumin, 44-45
    of serum osmolarity, 35-36
    tests in, 284-289
    of urea nitrogen, 36-37
    of urine osmolality, 37-38
    of urine pH, 42, 44
    of urine sodium, 39, *39t*
    of urine specific gravity, 38, *38t*
Lactase in enteral products, 252
Lactic acid, 44
Lactic acidosis, 172
    treatment of, 174-175
Laennec's cirrhosis, 233
Leukocytes, 7
Level of consciousness (LOC), changes
    in, 33-34
Long-chain triglycerides, 255
Lungs and fluid loss, 26

## M

Magnesium, 130-131
    foods high in, *133*

Magnesium—cont'd
    medications containing, *137*
    replacement for hypocalcemia,
        110-112
Magnesium balance disorders, 130-131
    hypermagnesemia
        assessment of, 136-137
        collaborative management of,
            137-138
        diagnostic tests for, 137
        nursing diagnoses and
            interventions for, 138-139
        patient-family teaching guidelines
            for, 139
    hypomagnesemia, 131
        assessment of, 131-132
        collaborative management of, 133
        diagnostic tests for, 132-133
        nursing diagnoses and
            interventions for, 133-135
        patient-family teaching guidelines
            for, 136
Malabsorption, 199
    as cause of hypomagnesemia, 131
Mechanical ventilation for metabolic
        acidosis, 174
Medium-chain triglycerides, 255
Membranes and movement of body
        fluids and solutes, 8
Metabolic acidosis, 79, 237
    acute, 170, 176t
        assessment of, 170, *171,* 172
        collaborative management of,
            173-174
        diagnostic tests for, 172-173,
            173t
        nursing diagnoses and
            interventions for, 175
    in acute adrenal insufficiency, 217
    in burns, 244
    in cardiogenic shock, 220
    causes of, *43*
    chronic, 175, 176t
        assessment of, 175
        collaborative management of, 177
        diagnostic tests for, 175, 177
        nursing diagnoses and
            interventions for, 177-178
    in congestive heart failure, 219
    in diabetic ketoacidosis, 206
    in gastrointestinal disorders, 200
    and hepatic failure, 236
    in hyperosmolar hyperglycemic non-
            ketotic syndrome, 207, 209
    as postoperative surgical
            disturbances, 203

Metabolic acidosis—cont'd
  potential causes of, *170*
  in pulmonary edema, 219
  in renal failure, 229
Metabolic alkalosis, 42, 79
  acute
    assessment of, 179-180
    collaborative management of,
      181-182
    diagnostic tests for, 181
    nursing diagnoses and
      interventions for, 182-183
  chronic
    assessment of, 183-184
    collaborative management of,
      184-185
    diagnostic tests for, 184
    nursing diagnoses and
      interventions for, 185
  in gastrointestinal disorders, 196
  and hepatic failure, 236
  potential causes of, *180*
Milk alkali syndrome, 184
Mixed acid-base disorders, case
  studies, 186-189
Mixed venous blood gases in metabolic
  acidosis, 172

**N**

Nausea, 34
Neurologic system, 33-34
Nitrogen balance studies, 248
Nonelectrolytes in body fluids, 6
Nursing assessment of patient at risk,
  27-34
Nursing diagnoses and interventions
  for acute metabolic acidosis, 175
  for acute metabolic alkalosis,
    182-183
  for acute respiratory acidosis,
    156-160
  for acute respiratory alkalosis,
    167-168
  for chronic metabolic acidosis,
    177-178
  for chronic metabolic alkalosis, 185
  for chronic respiratory acidosis,
    162-164
  for chronic respiratory alkalosis, 169
  for hypercalcemia, 115
  for hyperkalemia, 104-105
  for hypermagnesemia, 138-139
  for hypernatremia, 93-94
  for hyperphosphatemia, 127-129
  for hypervolemia, 70-72

Nursing diagnoses and interventions—
  cont'd
  for hypocalcemia, 110-112
  for hypokalemia, 99-101
  for hypomagnesemia, 133-135
  for hyponatremia, 90-91
  for hypophosphatemia, 122-124
  for hypovolemia, 65-67
Nursing history
  developmental, 27
  physiologic, 27
  psychologic, 28
  sociocultural, 28
  spiritual, 28
Nutrition; *see also* Diet
  altered, in metabolic acidosis,
    177-178
  estimating requirements in, 248
  sources of calcium in, *111*
  sources of magnesium in, *133*
  sources of phosphorus in, *121*
Nutritional support
  assessment in, 245
    anthropometric data, 246
    biochemical data, 247-250
    body mass index, 247
    height, 246
    history, 245-246
    physical, 246
    triceps skin fold thickness, 247
    weight, 246
  enteral, 250-253
    feeding tubes and sites in,
      251-252
    infusion rates in, 252, 252*t*
    managing complications in, 256,
      257-259*t*
    products in, 253, 254-255*t,* 255
  fluid requirements in, 250
  for hepatic failure, 249
  modalities, 250
  parenteral
    catheters in, 256, 260*t*
    monitoring infusion rates in, 256
    selection of feeding site in, 256
    solutions in, 260-261
  for renal disease, 250
  for respiratory disease, 250
  transitional feeding in, 261,
    263-264

**O**

Oliguria, 25
Oncotic pressure, 10
Oral fluids, 24, 29

Oral phosphates, 115
Oral rehydration in pediatric diarrhea, 55, 64*t*, 65
Osmolality, 11
  serum, 35-36
  urine, 37-38
Osmosis, 10-11
Osmotic diarrhea, *197,* 198-199
Osmotic diuresis, 10-11
Osmotic pressure, 10
Oxidative metabolism, 23-24
Oxygen therapy for management of respiratory acidosis, 162

**P**

Paco$_2$, 142
Pamidronate, 114
Pancreatic juice in gastrointestinal disorders, 198
Pancreatitis, acute
  potential fluid, electrolyte, and acid-base disturbances in, 230-232
  precipitating factors for, *231*
Pao$_2$, 142
Parathyroid hormone (PTH) secretion, 119
Parenteral nutrition
  in acute pancreatitis, 232
  catheters in, 256, 260*t*
  fluids in, 29
  managing complications in patients receiving, 262-263*t*
  monitoring infusion rates, 256
  selection of feeding site, 256
  solutions in, 260-261
Partial-thickness burns, 238
Patient-family teaching guidelines
  for hypercalcemia, 116-117
  for hyperkalemia, 106
  for hypermagnesemia, 139
  for hypernatremia, 94
  for hyperphosphatemia, 129
  for hypervolemia, 72-73
  for hypocalcemia, 112-113
  for hypokalemia, 101-102
  for hypomagnesemia, 136
  for hyponatremia, 91
  for hypophosphatemia, 124-125
  for hypovolemia, 67
Pediatric diarrhea, oral rehydration in, 55, 64*t*, 65
Peritoneal dialysis in management of chronic metabolic acidosis, 177
Peritonitis, 199

pH, 142
  urine, 42, 44
Pharmacotherapy for management of respiratory acidosis, 162
Phosphate, 4
  and acid-base balance, 141
  levels in chronic respiratory alkalosis, 169
Phosphorus, 118
  binding agents, 127*t*
  deficiency in, 119
  foods high in, *121*
  supplementation, 121
Phosphorus balance disorders, 118-119
  hyperphosphatemia as, 125
    assessment of, 125-126
    collaborative management of, 126-127, 127*t*
    diagnostic tests for, 126
    nursing diagnoses and interventions for, 127-129
    patient-family teaching guidelines for, 129
  hypophosphatemia as, 119
    assessment of, 119-121
    collaborative management of, *121,* 121-122
    diagnostic tests for, 121
    nursing diagnoses and interventions for, 122-124
    patient-family teaching guidelines for, 124-125
Physical assessment, 32
Platelets, 7
Plicamycin, 114
Polyuria, 11, 25
Postobstructive failure, 221
Postoperative ileus, risk or presence of, 203
Postrenal failure, 221
Potassium, 11
Potassium balance disorders, 95-96
  hyperkalemia as
    assessment of, 102-103
    collaborative management of, 103-104
    diagnostic tests for, 103
    nursing diagnoses and interventions for, 104-105
    patient-family teaching guidelines for, 106
  hypokalemia as, 96
    assessment of, 96-97
    collaborative management of, 97, 99
    diagnostic tests for, 97, *98*

Potassium balance disorders—cont'd
  hypokalemia as—cont'd
    nursing diagnoses and
        interventions for, 99-101
    patient-family teaching guidelines
        for, 101-102
Potassium replacement, 174
  in chronic metabolic alkalosis,
      184-185
Potassium-sparing diuretics in chronic
    metabolic alkalosis, 185
Prerenal failure, 221
Pressure
  oncotic, 10
  osmotic, 10
Prostaglandins, production of, in
    kidney, *222*
Protein
  and acid-base balance, 141
  in enteral products, 253, 255
  in parenteral solutions, 261
  status in measuring nutritional
      support, 247
Pulmonary artery pressure (PAP), 30
Pulmonary edema; *see* Edema

# R

Red blood cells (RBCs), 7, 36
Renal disease, 170
  diet for, 250
Renal failure, 36
  acute, 221-222
    causes of, 223-224*t*
    treatment of, 174
  chronic, 226
  drugs that require dosage
      modification in, 225*t*
  potential fluid, electrolyte, and
      acid-base disturbances,
      226-229, *227, 228*
Renal system, buffer response of, 141
Renal tubular acidosis
  in acute adrenal insufficiency, 217
  treatment of, 174
Renal tubules, 10
Renin, production of, in kidney, *222*
Renin-angiotensin, 15
Respiratory acidosis, 237, 244
  acute, 153
    assessment of, 153-155, *154*
    collaborative management of, 155
    diagnostic tests for, 155
    nursing diagnoses and
        interventions for, 156-160
  in burns, 244

Respiratory acidosis—cont'd
  chronic
    assessment of, 160-161, *161*
    collaborative management of, 162
    diagnostic tests for, 161-162
    nursing diagnoses and
        interventions for, 162-164
  in congestive heart failure, 219
  diet for, 264
  as postoperative surgical
      disturbances, 203
  in pulmonary edema, 219
Respiratory alkalosis, 118-119, 120
  acute
    assessment of, 165-166
    collaborative management of, 167
    diagnostic tests for, 166-167
    nursing diagnoses and
        interventions for, 167-168
  in acute pancreatitis, 232
  in burns, 244
  chronic
    assessment of, 168
    collaborative management of, 169
    diagnostic tests for, 168
    nursing diagnoses and
        interventions for, 169
  in congestive heart failure, 219
  and hepatic failure, 236
  as postoperative surgical
      disturbances, 203
  in pulmonary edema, 219
Respiratory disease, diet for, 250
Respiratory rate, rapid or labored, 29
Respiratory rate and depth, 31
Respiratory system, buffer response of,
    141
Restlessness, 34
Reye's syndrome, 233

# S

Sacral edema, 74
Saliva in gastrointestinal disorders,
    193, 195
Secretory diarrhea, *197, 199*
Sensible fluid, 25
Serum albumin, 44-45
Serum electrolytes
  in acute metabolic alkalosis, 181
  in acute respiratory acidosis, 155
  in acute respiratory alkalosis,
      166-167
  in chronic metabolic acidosis, 175
  in chronic metabolic alkalosis, 184
  in chronic respiratory alkalosis, 168

Serum electrolytes—cont'd
  in hypovolemia, 52-53
  in metabolic acidosis, 172
  normal ranges, 40t
Serum osmolality, 35-36
  in hypovolemia, 53
Serum phosphate in acute respiratory
    alkalosis, 167
Serum potassium in hyperkalemia, 103
Serum sodium for hypervolemia, 69
Serum total carbon dioxide in
    hypovolemia, 53
Shock, hypovolemic, 49
Short bowel syndrome, 197
Simple diffusion, 9
Skin and fluid loss, 25
Skin turgor, 32
Small bowel as feeding tube site,
    251-252
Sodium, 11
Sodium balance disorders
  changes, 87-88
  hypernatremia as
    assessment of, 91-92
    collaborative management of, 93
    diagnostic tests for, 92-93
    nursing diagnoses and
      interventions for, 93-94
    patient-family teaching guidelines
      for, 94
  hyponatremia as, 88
    assessment of, 88-89
    collaborative management of, 89
    diagnostic tests for, 89
    with expanded extracellular fluid
      volume, 90
    nursing diagnoses and
      interventions for, 90-91
    patient-family teaching guidelines
      for, 91
    with reduced extracellular fluid
      volume, 89-90
Sodium overload, 36
Solid foods, 24
Solutes
  in body fluids, 4, 5t, 6
  factors that affect movement of, 8-13
Sputum culture in chronic respiratory
    acidosis, 162
Stomach as feeding tube site, 251
Surgical disturbances, 201-203
  intraoperative factors in, 202
  postoperative factors in, 202-203
  preoperative factors in, 201
Sweating, 25
  excessive, 29

Sympathetic nervous system, 15, 18
Syndrome of inappropriate antidiuretic
    hormone (SIADH), 36, 215
  potential fluid, electrolyte, and
    acid-base disturbances in,
    215
Systemic vascular resistance (SVR), 31

**T**

Third space fluid, 202
  disorders associated with shift, 50t
Third-space fluid shift, 26
Third-space losses and fluid loss, 26
Thirst, 20, 21-22, 34
  and antidiuretic hormone, 21
Thrombocytopenia, 233
Thyroxine-binding albumin, 247
Tissue integrity, impaired, in
    hypervolemia, 72
Tonicity, 12
Total $CO_2$, 40-41
  in acute metabolic alkalosis, 181
  in acute respiratory acidosis, 155
  in chronic metabolic acidosis, 175
  in chronic metabolic alkalosis, 184
  in chronic respiratory acidosis, 161
  in metabolic acidosis, 172
Total nutrient admixtures (TNA),
    260-261
Transcellular fluid (TCF) in body
    fluids, 7-8
Transferrin, 247
Transfusion reactions, 81
  acute, 82-84t
Transitional feeding, 261, 263-264
Transport processes and movement of
    body fluids and solutes, 8-13
Triceps skin fold thickness, 247
Trousseau's sign, positive, 34
  in assessing hyperphosphatemia, 128
  in assessing hypocalcemia, 108
Tube feedings, 29
Tubular necrosis in cardiogenic shock,
    220

**U**

Ulcerative colitis, 199
Urea nitrogen, 36-37
Urinary output, normal, 25
Urinary sodium for hypervolemia, 69
Urine, concentration of, 24-25
Urine osmolality, 37-38
Urine pH, 42, 44
Urine potassium in hyperkalemia, 103

Urine sodium, 39, 39t
  in hypovolemia, 53
Urine specific gravity, 38, 38t
  in hypervolemia, 69
  in hypovolemia, 53


V

Vascular volume, regulation of,
  14-15, 18
Vital signs, 30
Vitamin D therapy for hypocalcemia,
  110

Volume abnormalities and diuretic
  therapy, 75
Vomiting, 34
  potential causes of, 195


W

Water
  in body fluids, 3-4, 4t
  factors that affect movement of, 8-13
Weight, 246
White blood cells (WBC), 7
Wound drainage, 29